The ABCs of Extrapelvic Endometriosis

EXTRAPELVIC NOT RARE
where science meets community

Wendy Bingham DPT
Extrapelvic Not Rare 501(c)(3)

Title: The ABCs of Extrapelvic Endometriosis

Author: Wendy Bingham DPT
Published by Wendy Bingham DPT, Vancouver, WA. USA

Requests permission to use content:
Wendy Bingham DPT
Extrapelvic Not Rare (501 c3)
wendybinghamdpt@extrapelvicnotrare.org

Thank you to the following individuals whose voluntary services have contributed to the production this book:

Editing and Proofread: Holly Dandurand, Ken Dandurand, Alexandra Mitchell
Graphic design, cover and content layout: Kelli Cerruto
Translations: Natalia Forero (Spanish), Martina Liel (German), Sarah Méric-Ducos (French), Sarah Yvonne Ramos (Spanish)

Illustrations and Photo Images provided through Canva.com

Available Languages: English, French, German, Spanish
Content of this book is supported by documented, histologically confirmed endometriosis (tissue samples) among each physiological structure. Each location is reported once or more in scientific literature (see citations at end of book).

ISBN 979-8-9901141-4-2

Library of Congress 2025900473

*This book is intended to be inclusive of all persons with endometriosis. The use of the word woman and/or female refers to the assigned sex at birth, however gender identity can differ than the assigned sex at birth.

Content

Preface....................v-vii
Introduction....................viii-xii
Book Layout....................xiii
Definitions....................xiv-viii

Section I
Did You Know?....................1-11
Endometriosis
the disease....................2-3
adhesions....................3
who develops it....................4-5
symptoms....................5-6
young adults....................7
comorbidites....................7-8
autoimmune diseases....................8
extrapelvic....................9-10
complications....................10-11

Section II
Extrapelvic Endometriosis: A to Z in Pictures..........13
A to Z Colour Images....................14-106
What is Extrapelvic Not Rare?....................108
Citations....................109-154
Did You Know?....................110-129
A to Z Picture Library....................130-154

Preface

Over the past century, disease beyond the reproductive organs and true pelvis has been routinely reported, though at times infrequent. The internet era has rapidly expanded the number of available journals and access to them; giving rise to an exponential growth in the number of confirmed cases of disease that do not fit the established profile of endometriosis.

The International Classification of Diseases (ICD) is the most widely used system to document each incident of endometriosis. Prior to 2022 (ICD-11) the option to record each occurrence of disease beyond the reproductive areas was limited to a few places. Revision of the 10th version expanded these options. At time of publication, the number and detail of locations available includes, but is not limited to, the cecum, appendix, bladder, ureter and diaphragm. This is a step forward.

The statements in this book are facts. These facts are supported by evidence. This evidence challenges the long established disease profile known to those who practice medicine, conduct research, and provide content on media platforms.

The idea for this book began nearly eight years ago. I was curious if locations of endometriosis (histologically confirmed) could be identified for each letter of the English alphabet. Over the intervening years the number of locations has grown, and with it, the amount of data about the disease. Published reports and personal experiences of countless individuals with endometriosis in areas of the body other than, or in addition to, the reproductive area, have inspired the development of this book.

We, the people with endometriosis, are keenly aware of the disparity between living with the disease and the established profile that healthcare professionals, their governing bodies and research scientists use to guide their decisions.

As a licensed medical practitioner who has endometriosis, I have a perspective of the disease through the lens of those who provide medical care and those who receive it. The disparity between perspectives is significant.

The hallmark symptom, painful menstruation (periods), is not regularly experienced by all persons with endometriosis.

Some have infrequent and/or less intense pain during menstruation (dysmenorrhea). Others never experience pain pain during menstruation.

Far too many people also endure long diagnostic delays, whether or not they experience 'bad periods'. Those with severe dysmenorrhea are often accused of exaggerating their symptoms or told they "can't have endometriosis." Patients with cyclical symptoms not directly associated with menstruation are often dismissed or misdiagnosed for another condition, with endometriosis rarely considered.

Failure to understand the disease and recognize all possible symptoms and complications, alters the trajectory of people's lives. Delayed diagnosis often leads to complications and irreversible damage. To reiterate, the damage is **NOT** limited to reproductive tissues. Endometriosis can damage other body systems and disrupt their functions.

I hope this book educates, inspires and broadens your own view of this complicated disease and its widespread affects.

- Wendy Bingham, DPT

Introduction

This book is about endometriosis. It has two purposes. The first purpose is to provide evidence that challenges the perception of endometriosis as a simple disease.

Throughout history, with exception to a few societies of limited duration, people born female have faced prejudices that have, and continue to diminish their position as inferior to those born male. The perception women* are inferior to men (mentally, emotionally and physically) is directly responsible for the chasm between what is known about diseases that predominantly or exclusively affect persons born female* to those born male.

Hence, by way of historical association, endometriosis has been plagued with preconceived notions since it was first identified.

Until recent years, endometriosis has been simplified to a disease with destructive capacity limited to the reproductive areas of people who are born, and identify as cis-female during the years of menstruation, with symptoms limited to days actively menstruating, the misconception that endometriosis can be cured with pregnancy, hormone suppression therapy or removal of the uterus (hysterectomy) with or without the ovaries (oophorectomy) persists despite abundant evidence to refute these claims.

The book's second purpose is to serve as a resource for persons who identify with the content provided in these pages; whether already diagnosed or seeking a diagnosis for symptoms whose source has yet to be identified.

The reproductive area is not the only place endometriosis occurs. While it is the most common area affected by the disease, it has been found among all the major organs of the human body and systems they are part of (except taste, sight, and hearing).

Accumulating evidence and experiences of persons with the disease are generating an uptick of interest in endometriosis. The shift from the simplified view of how endometriosis has always been understood, to a highly complex disease is long overdue. It is imperative that any disease profile be fluid and evolve from **all** available evidence, not just what fits specific theory(ies) of origin(s), diagnostics or intervention(s).

Endometriosis is not simple. It is a complex disease that can disrupt a wide range of systemic functions. It often occurs with other health conditions and can occur anywhere in the body.

No two people experience endometriosis exactly the same way. However, some common symptoms are experienced in a high percentage of people.

The presence of endometriosis, regardless of location, often contributes to symptoms from non-reproductive organs. Common examples include gastrointestinal symptoms such as bloating, diarrhea and constipation; urinary symptoms such as the frequent need to empty the bladder that may be painful; thigh pain and migraine headaches.

The extrapelvic locations included in this book are gathered from online databases of articles published in English. The number of persons reported for each location range from one person to upwards of millions. For example, based on this author's investigation, some locations have only been reported once (e.g. thumb).

Other locations range from a handful (nose), less than a dozen (ie. spleen), a few dozen (ie. liver body) and so forth. The frequeny of disease insome locations are in the millions; of which published cases are a very small representation (ie. rectum, bladder).

Most, but not all locations of extrapelvic endometriosis present with symptoms pertaining to the involved organ. For example, persons with endometriosis of the rectum may experience the same gastrointestinal symptoms, but more intense and with additional concerns (ie. severe pain and/or blood with bowel movements, history of bowel obstructions).

Some locations, such as the brain, have only been reported in the literature a handful of times. Persons diagnosed with endometriosis, and who experience migraine headaches, should not immediately suspect they have endometriosis of the brain. The probability is tiny. However, one can never say never.

Journaling your symptoms provides useful information for your healthcare team. Important items to include:

- **When** symptom(s) occur. Do they appear or disappear with your menstrual cycle or at certain times of the day?

- What do the symptoms feel like?
- Where do you feel symptoms?
- Do specific movements, positions, foods, medications, heat or cold affect symptoms?

This book was created to affirm common and scarcely known facts about the disease and those affected by it. It dispels the stereotype of endometriosis as a simple disease, confined to reproductive areas that has long shaped the direction of research and care for people with this disease.

Awareness inspires conversations.

Conversations build knowledge.

Knowledge drives actions.

Actions transform.

Let's get started.

Book Layout

The content of this book has been organized to easily locate information. It is divided into two sections. The first section opens with definitions, and a few diagrams. This is followed by “Did You Know?”

“Did You Know?” provides general information about endometriosis that is organized by topic. Each topic contains concise, referenced bullet point facts for easy access to discuss and share content with others, including your healthcare team.

The second section contains images of locations where **extrapelvic** endometriosis has been documented. Locations are organized A to Z based upon their names in English.

Pelvic endometriosis is specific to the female reproductive system; located in the true pelvis (the lower portion on the bony pelvis). Hence, endometriosis of the male reproductive system is included in this book as extrapelvic.

Endometriosis: The Definitions

Tomassetti C, Johnson NP, Petrozza J, Abrao MS, Einarsson JI, et al. 2021

Endometriosis is "a disease characterized by the presence of endometrium-like epithelium and/or stroma outside the endometrium and myometrium (uterus),"

An International Terminology for Endometriosis, International Working Group of AAGL, ESGE, ESHRE and WES. JMIG.2021;28(11).
Doi: 10.1016/j.jmig.2021.08.032

Endometriosis: Definitions

Markam (1987, 1989, 1991, 1997)

Pelvic endometriosis is defined as endometriotic lesions involving the (outer) uterus, fallopian tubes, ovaries and the surrounding peritoneum, the anterior and posterior cul-de-sac and pelvic sidewalls.

Extrapelvic endometriosis is described as endometriotic-like lesions elsewhere in the body.

Jubanyik and Comite (1997)

As in earlier articles (ref), pelvic endometriosis is defined as lesions of the fallopian tubes, ovaries, and local peritoneum. Extrapelvic endometriosis refers to endometriotic implants found elsewhere in the body, including the gastrointestinal tract, urinary tract, pulmonary system, extremities, skin, and central nervous system (CNS).

Endometriosis: Definitions

Yazdanian et al. (2014)

Extrapelvic endometriosis is defined as the presence of endometriotic lesions found outside the pelvis and elsewhere in the body including the

- cervix
- vagina
- vulva
- intestinal tract
- urinary tract
- diaphragm
- abdominal wall
- inguinal canal
- thoracic cage
- lungs
- limbs
- central and peripheral nervous systems

Learn more about extrapelvic endometriosis:
www.extrapelvicnotrare.org

Pelvic Endometriosis

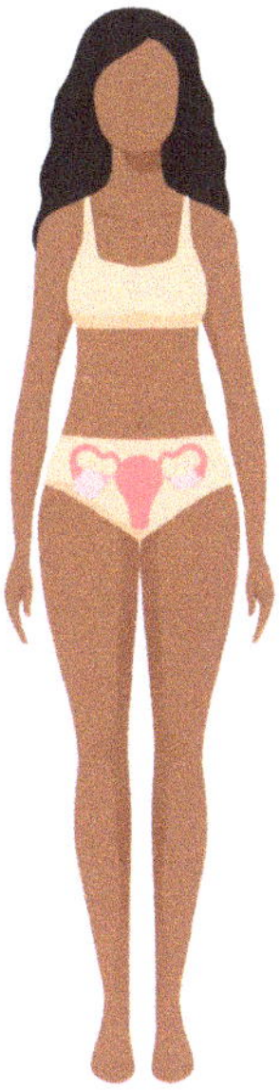

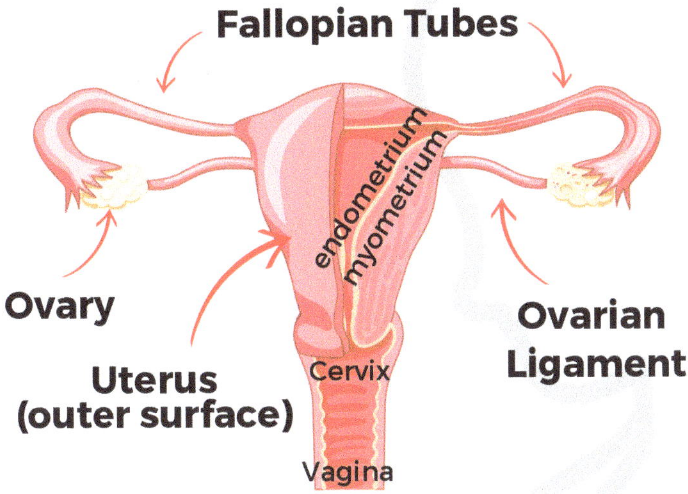

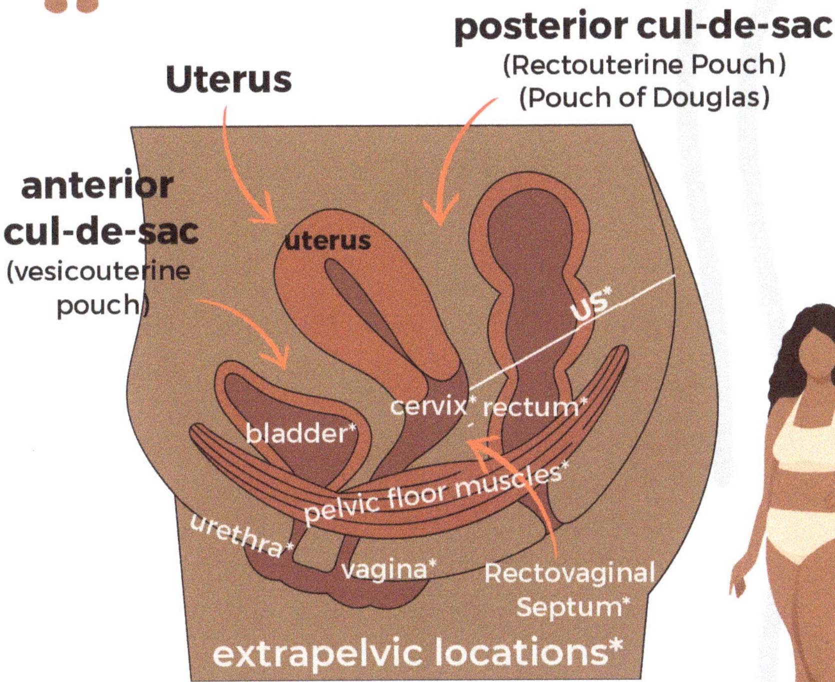

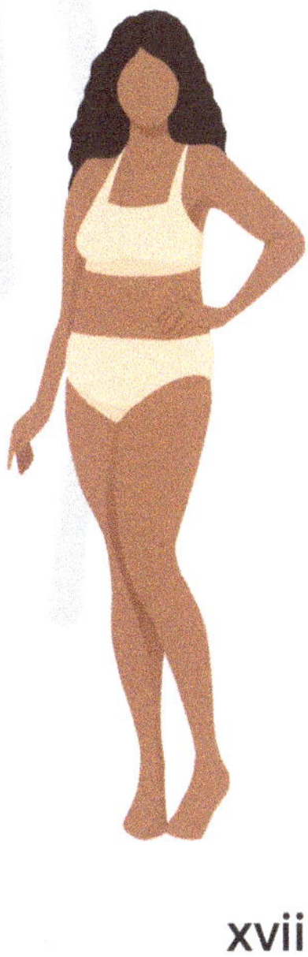

<u>**not pictured**</u>
pelvic sidewalls
uterine ligaments:
Broad, Round, Uterosacral

Extrapelvic Endometriosis:

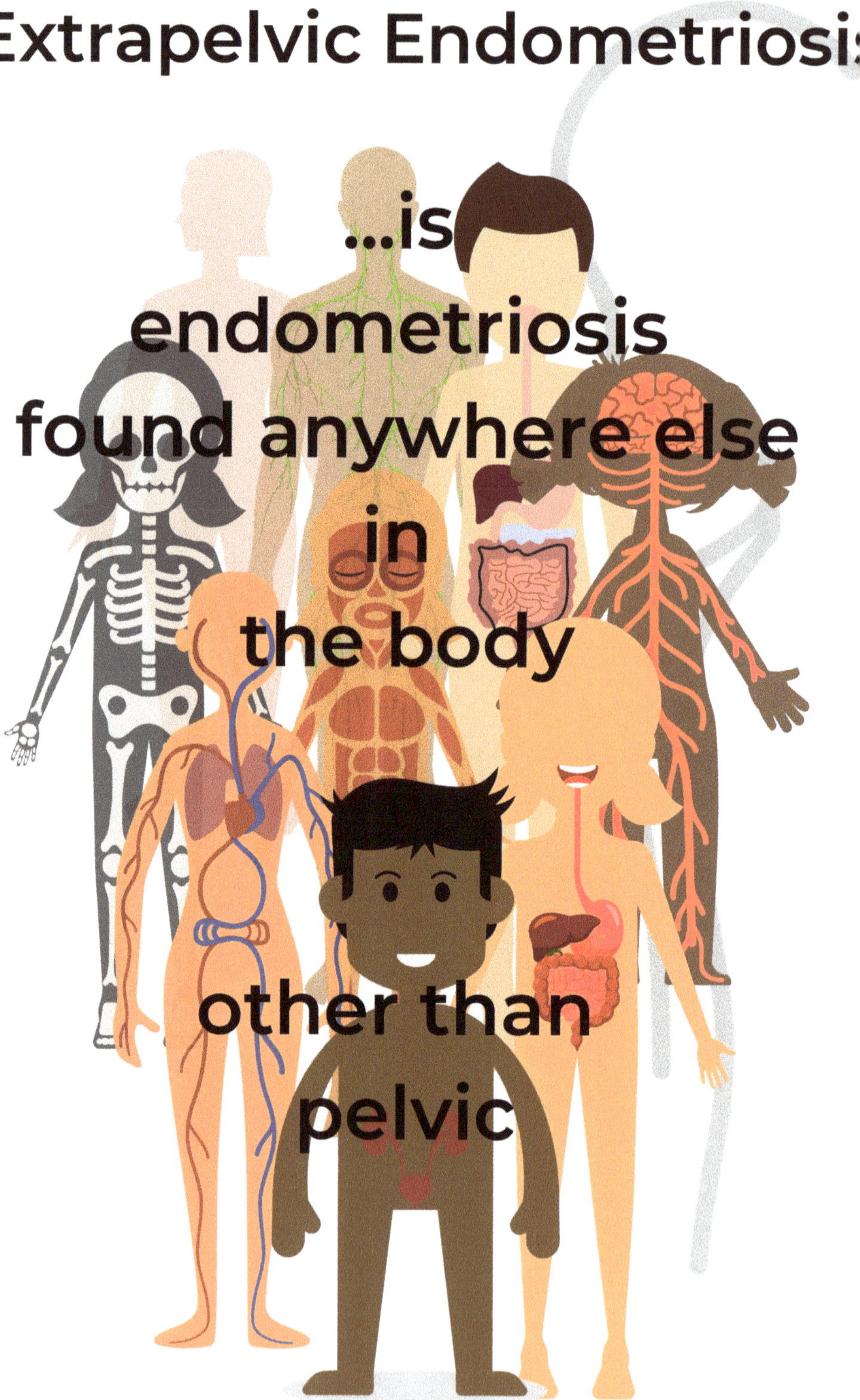

...is endometriosis found anywhere else in the body other than pelvic

Section I

Did You Know?

Endometriosis

Did You Know?

Endometriosis: the disease

...appears grossly similar to the inner lining of the uterus but possess unique properties. (1,2)

...lesions are also called 'foci' and 'implants'. (2,3)

...lesions are initially comprised of glands and/or stroma. Lesion composition may change as the disease progresses. (2-4)

...lesions occur in different shapes and colours. The type of cells, age and activity contribute to each lesion's appearance. (2,4-8)

...is influenced by the same hormones that cause menstruation, (the regular shedding of the inner lining of the uterus about every month). These hormones are estrogen and progesterone. (2,3)

...causes inflammation in areas of lesions (local) and contributes to body-wide inflammation (systemic). (9)

...is not an autoimmune disease, but commonly occurs with one or more. (10)

Did You Know?

Endometriosis: the disease

...lesions interfere with the immune system's ability to breakdown and remove lesion debri. This contributes to persistent, chronic inflammation in addition to recurrent acute episodes that coincide menstruation. (1,11)

Endometriosis: adhesions

...are the result of lesion activity and the immune system's attempt to clear the body of 'foreign debri' (foreign by location & product). (12)

...adhesions bind two or more surfaces together (ie. bladder to uterus, uterus to colon, diaphragm to liver, ovary to pelvic sidewall, intestine to abdominal wall) and can develop blood vessels and nerves. (12-14)

...adhesions can restrict normal organ movement and function. (ie. Adhesions can impair the passage of food waste from the body and urine to drain from the kidney to the bladder.) (12,14)

Did You Know?

Endometriosis: who develops it

...affects an estimated 1 in 10 people born female. (15)

...occurs in people who menstruate, no longer menstruate or have never menstruated. (16)

...occurs among people who identify as female, agender, non-binary, transgender and (rare) cis-males. (17,18)

...can begin before the first menses (menarche). (19)

...can occur in people born without a uterus, and onset or persist after it is removed. (20,21)

...has been diagnosed in people as young as 7, and over 90 yrs of age. (22,23)

...can begin or remain active after menopause, even if hormone replacement therapy has never been used. (22,23)

Did You Know?

Endometriosis: who develops it

...is documented among aborted female fetuses, primates, and non-human mammals such as dogs, guinea pigs and cows. (24-26)

Note: Humans, primates, and shrews menstruate. All other mammals do not menstruate. Non-menstruating mammals are anestrus. (24-26)

Endometriosis: symptoms

...according to publications, the average delay to diagnosis is 6.6 years. One study reported a range of 11.3 yrs (USA) and 1.5 yrs (Australia).(27)

...symptoms (most commonly) begin to appear on the days leading up to, and through menses. (28,29)

...disease progression is associated with an incremental rise in the number of days per month symptoms are present. (29)

Did You Know?

Endometriosis: symptoms

...symptoms include, but are not limited to: (27,28)

- severe pain with menstruation
- abdominal bloating and cramping,
- diarrhea, constipation or cycling of both
- pain with bowel movements or urination
- painful sex
- unable to conceive (become pregnant).

...can also cause:

- a generally unwell feeling
- fatigue not resolved with a good night's sleep
- muscle and joint pain
- high blood cholesterol
- and more due to inflammation.

...symptoms are also determined by the organ or tissue the lesion(s) are among or near. (29-32)

Did You Know?

Endometriosis: young adults

...occurs more often among those with symptoms and/or diagnosis of Irritable Bowel Syndrome (IBS). (33,34)

...< 20 yrs of age with endometriosis are > 5x more likely to have symptoms or diagnosis of IBS than those without endometriosis. (34)

...occurs more often among those with a history of migraine headaches. (35)

...may have symptoms that are present on days other than menstruation. (36)

Endometriosis: comorbidities

...conditions that often co-occur (10,33-35,37-41):

- Allergies (environmental and food)
- Asthma*
- Cardiovascular Disease (CVD)*
- Chronic Fatigue Syndrome (ME/CFS)
- Fibromyalgia
- Interstitial Cystitis (IC)
- Irritable Bowel Syndrome
- Mast Cell Disorders

* overlap of common genetic expression with endometriosis

Did You Know?

Endometriosis: comorbidities

- Migraine Headaches*
- Postural Orthostatic Tachycardia Syndrome (POTS)

* overlap of common genetic expression with endometriosis

Endometriosis: autoimmune diseases

...autoimmune conditions reported to have an association or genetic relationship (11,39,42,43):

- Addison's Disease
- Ankylosing Spondylitis (AS)
- Celiac Disease
- Connective Tissue Disorders
  - Rheumatoid Arthritis (RA)
  - Sjorgen's Syndrome, Systemic Lupus Erythematosus (SLE).
- Hashimoto's Disease
- Inflammatory Bowel Diseasse (IBD)
  - Chrohn's Disease (CD)
  - Ulcerative Colitis (UC)
- Multiple Sclerosis (MS)

Note: Ehlers-Danlos, Marfan's and Loeys-Dietz Syndromes are hereditary connective tissue disorders reported in persons with endometriosis. At time of publication the quantity of quality studies were available to declare any relation between endometriosis and these conditions.

Did You Know?

Endometriosis: extrapelvic

...an estimated 20% to 37% of people with pelvic endometriosis also have disease in extrapelvic areas. (44-46)

(Note: estimates are based upon publications prior to the 2022 revisions of the International Classification of Diseases (10th Version).

...the **digestive system** is the most common location for endometriosis outside the reproductive area. Lesions most frequently affect the large intestine, particularly the rectum and sigmoid colon. (45,47,48)

...the **urinary system** is the second most common location for endometriosis outside the reproductive area. Lesions most frequently affect the bladder. (47,48)

...the **respiratory system** is the third most common location for endometriosis outside the reproductive area. Lesions most frequently affect the diaphragm. (46)

Did You Know?

Endometriosis: extrapelvic

...Skin layers (cutaneous system) are estimated the fourth most common extrapelvic system. Primary lesions affect intact areas and secondary lesions affect surgical scars. The belly button (umbilicus) is most common site. (47,49)

...a few extrapelvic locations are frequently asymptomatic (ie. kidney) or symptoms do not adhere to the cyclic pattern that peaks during menstruation (ie. liver and pancreas). (50,51)

Endometriosis: complications

... Endometriosis is present in up to 50% of individuals who unable to conceive (become pregnant) naturally and/or are high risk pregnancies. (15,52,53) These include:

- who have symptoms that suggest the presence of endometrieosis
- who have a diagnosis of endometriosis and are symptomatic.
- who have no symptoms but have an endometriosis diagnosis
- who have no symptoms or a diagnosis of endometriosis with 'unexplained' infertility

Did You Know?
Endometriosis: complications

...extrapelvic endometriosis can cause:

- blood in stool (hematochezia) (54-56)
- bowel blockage (obstruction) (57-59)
- bowel incontinence (60,61)
- kidney damage/death (hydronephrosis) (62,63)
- blood in urine (hematouria) (64,65)
- urinary retention (65,66)
- urinary incontinence (65,66)
- lung collapse (pneumothorax) (67-70)
- fluid w/wo blood in the chest (pleural effusion or hemothorax) (71-74)
- cough of blood (hemoptysis) (75,76)
- diaphragm herniation (71,72)
- neuropathy (peripheral - ie. foot drop) (77,78)

...and more.

Section II

Extrapelvic Endometriosis

A to Z in Pictures

A

Adductors (muscle group)

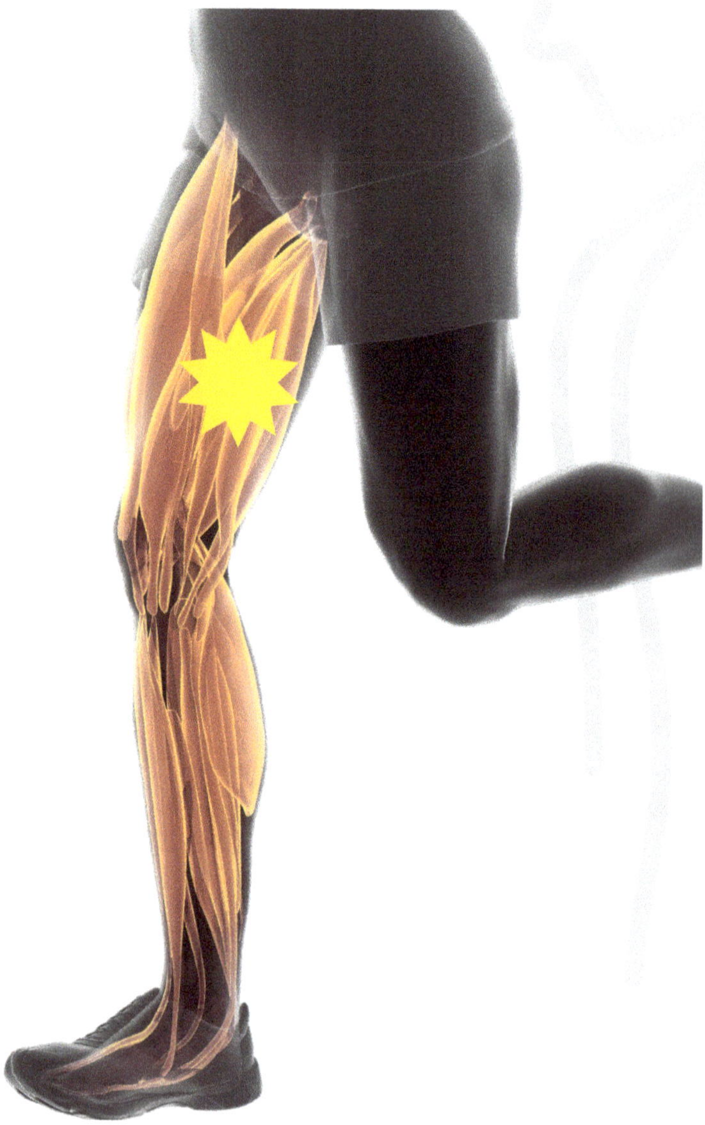

A

Adrenal Gland

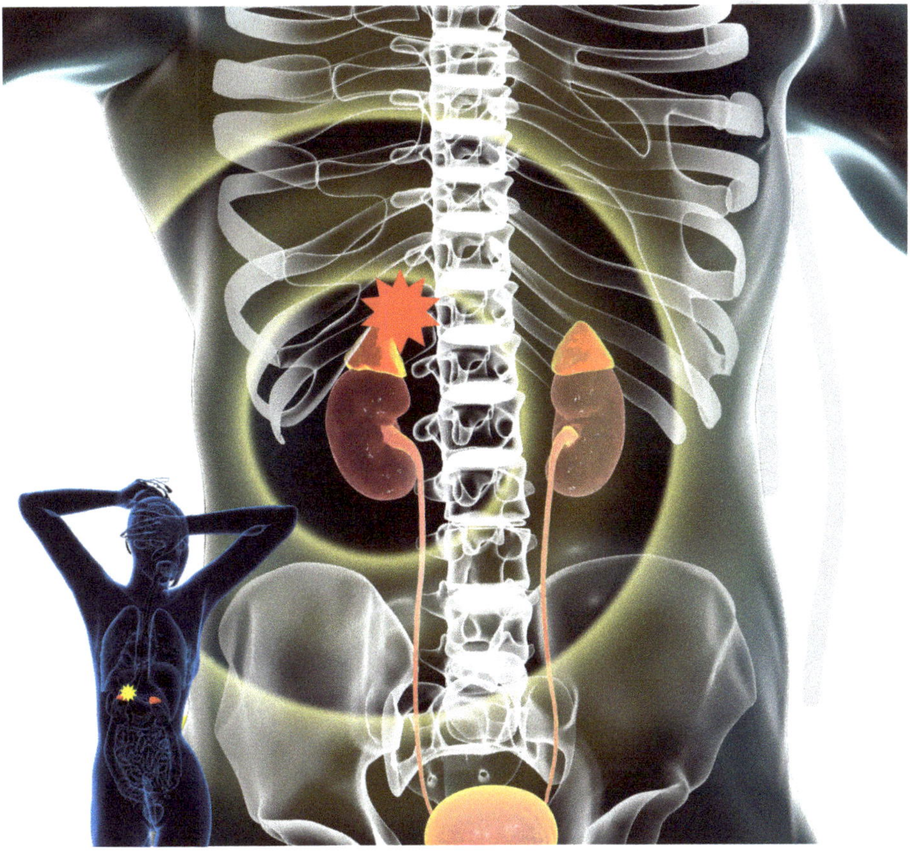

A

Alcock's Canal

(not pictured)

Alveoli

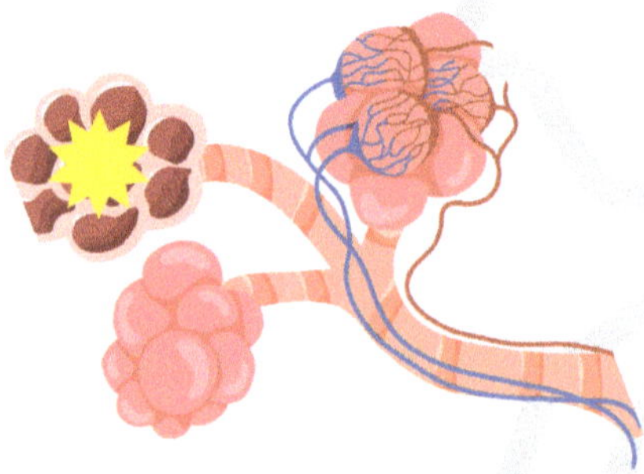

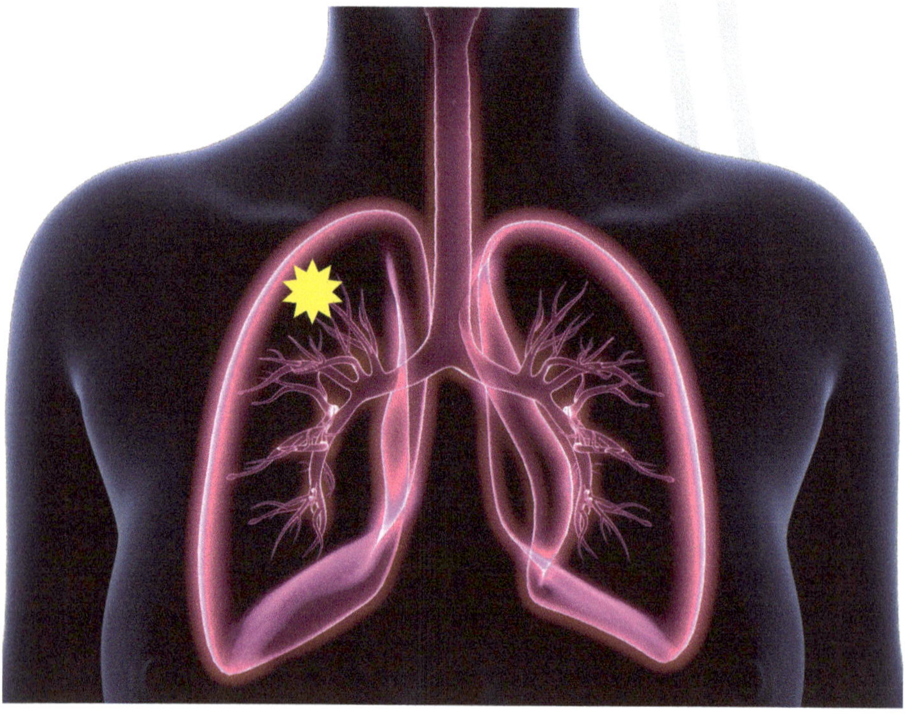

A

Aorta (thoracic)

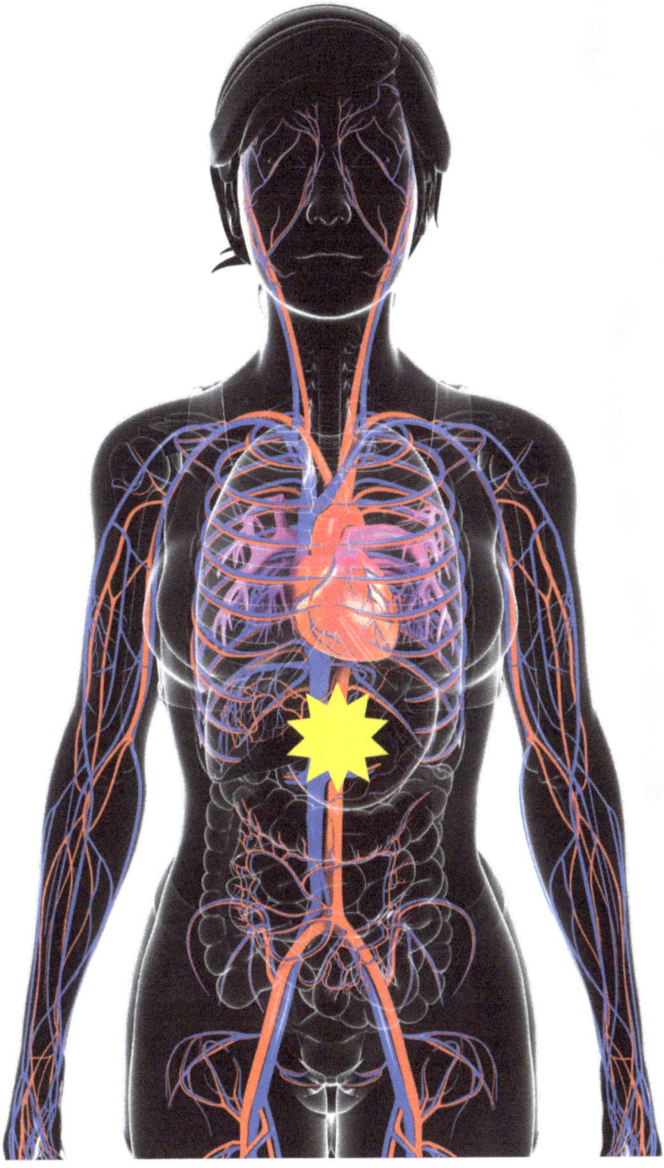

A

Appendix

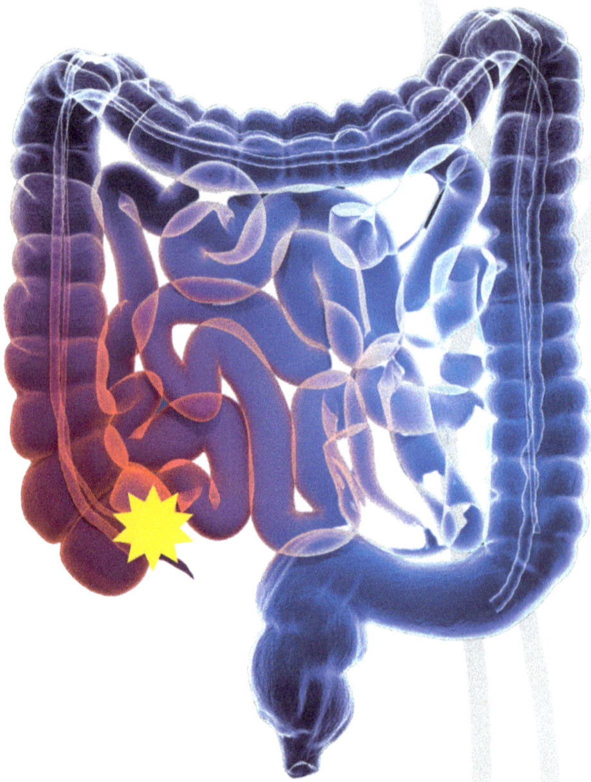

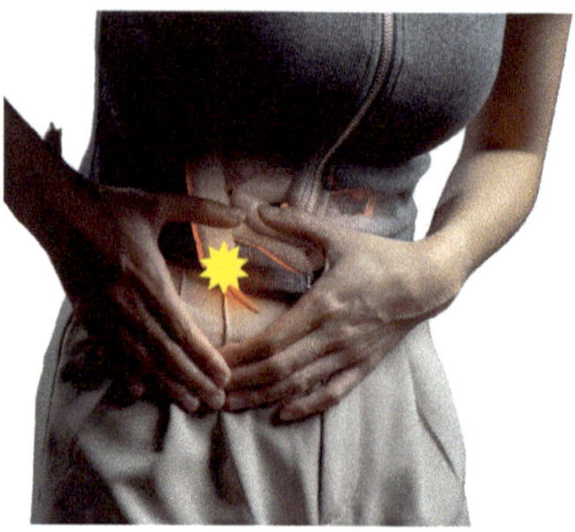

A

Ascending Colon

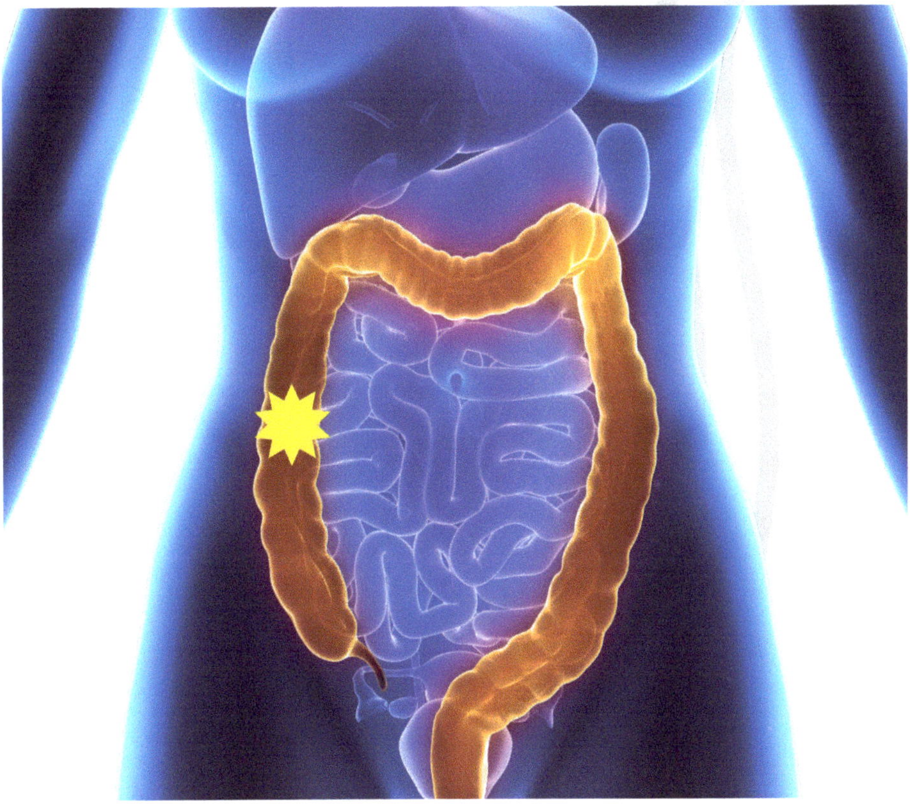

B

Biceps Femoris (muscle)

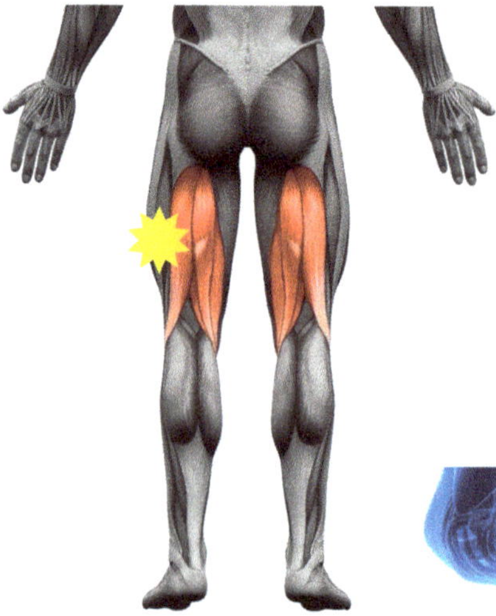

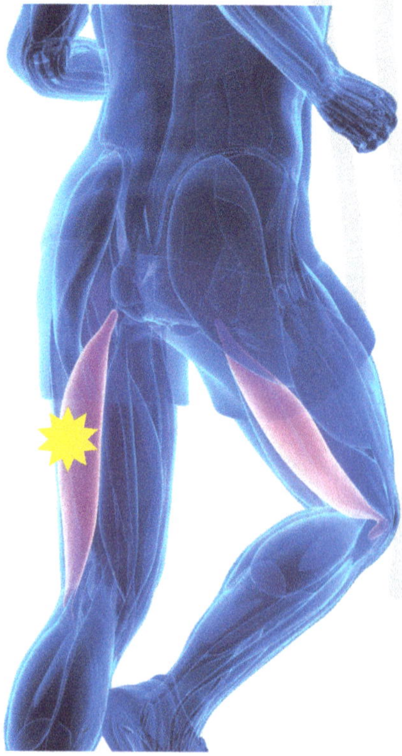

B
Bladder

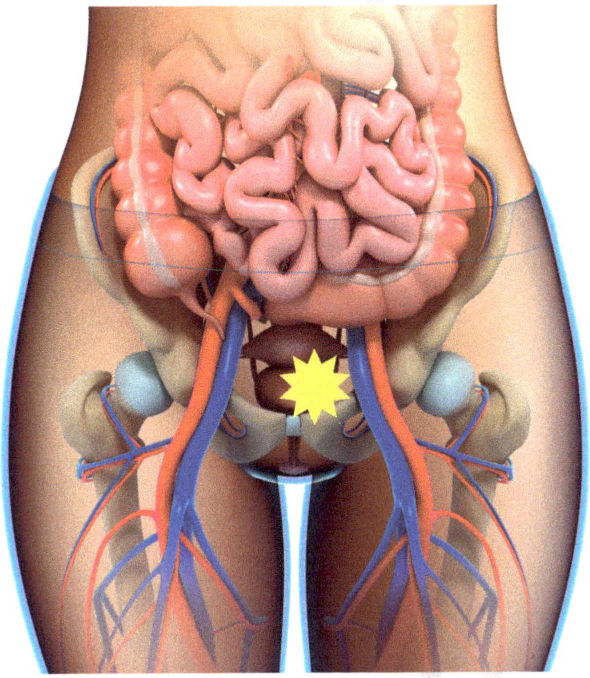

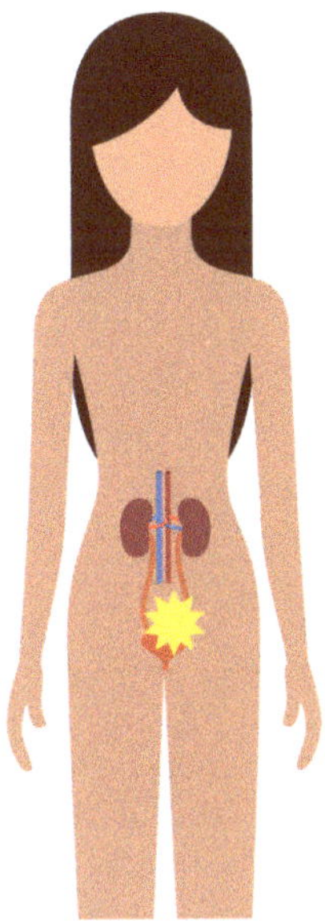

B

Bone

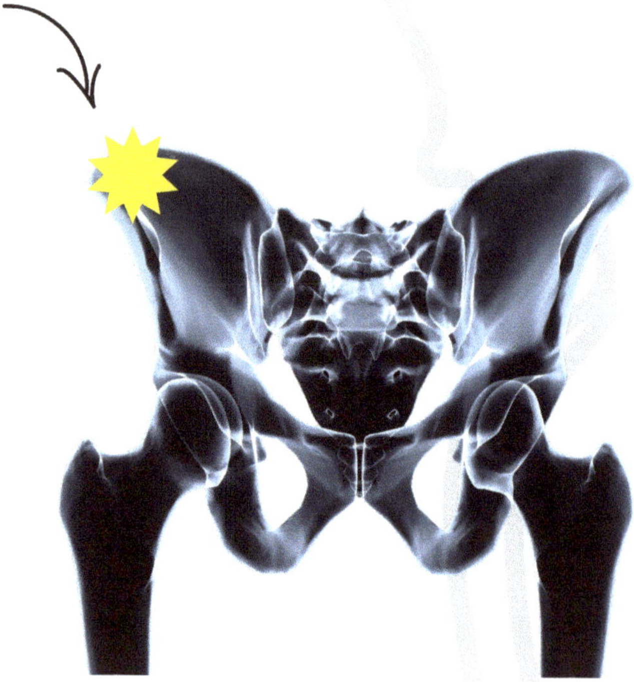

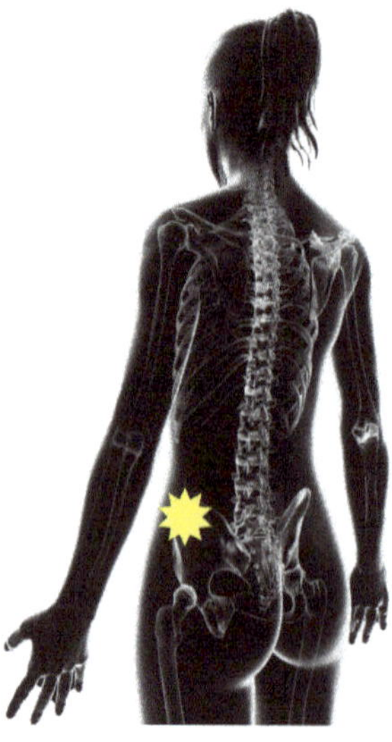

B

Brachioradialis (muscle)

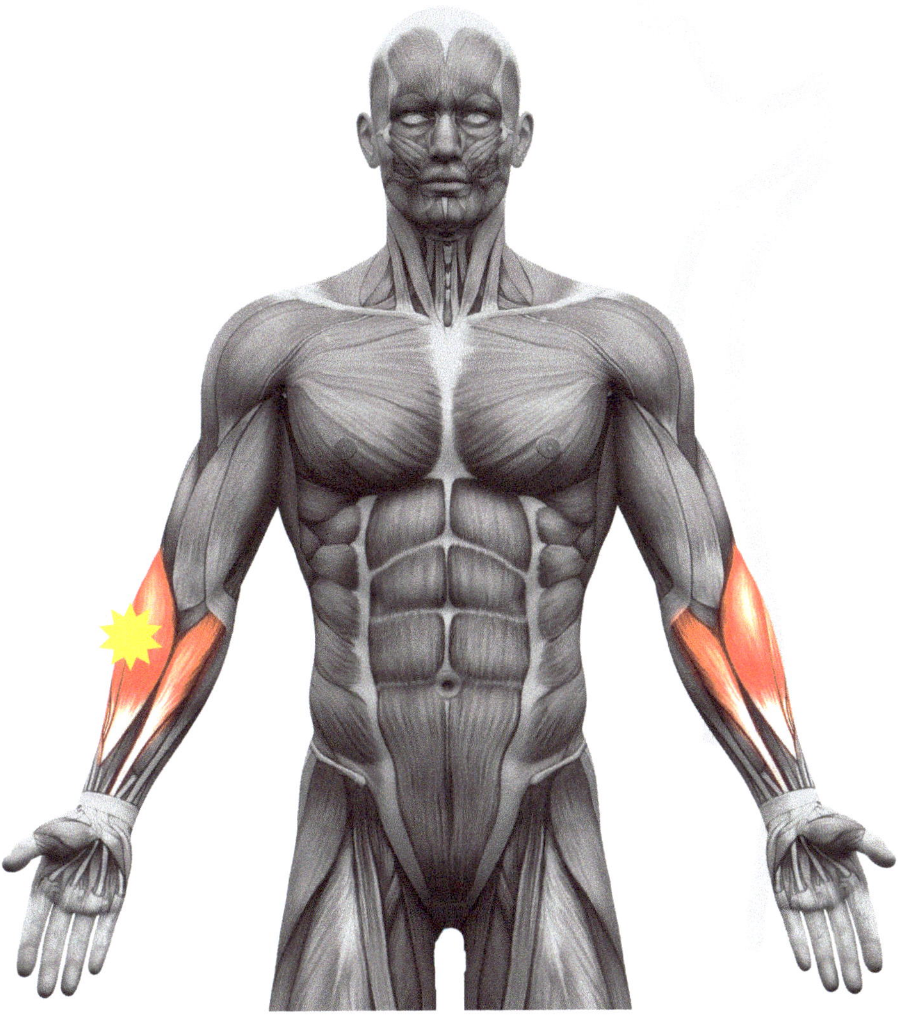

B

Breast

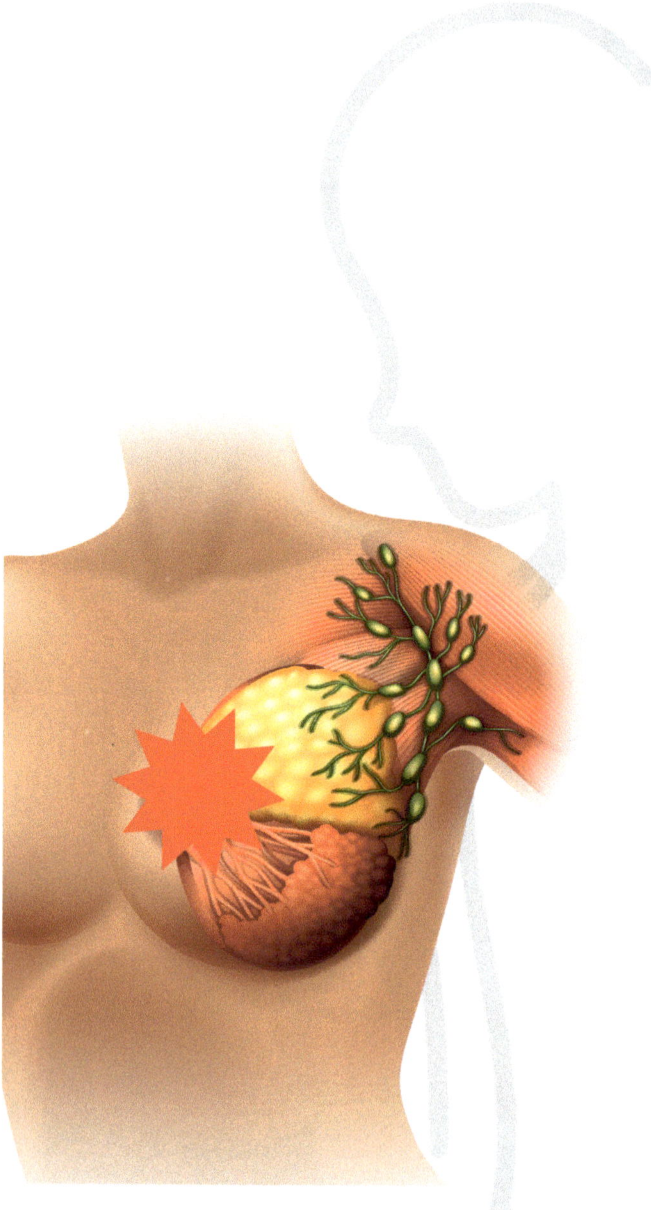

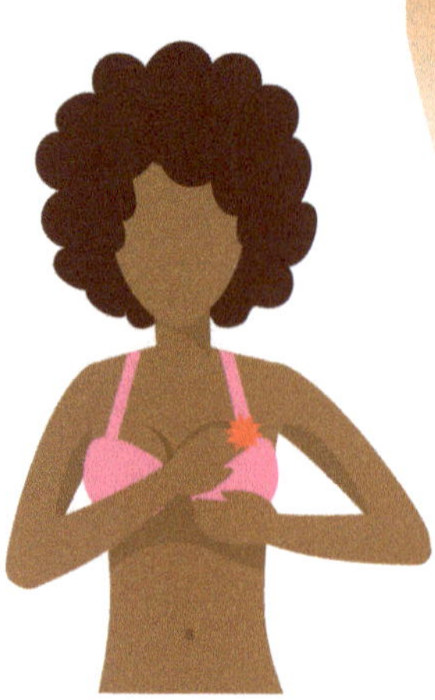

B
Bronchiole

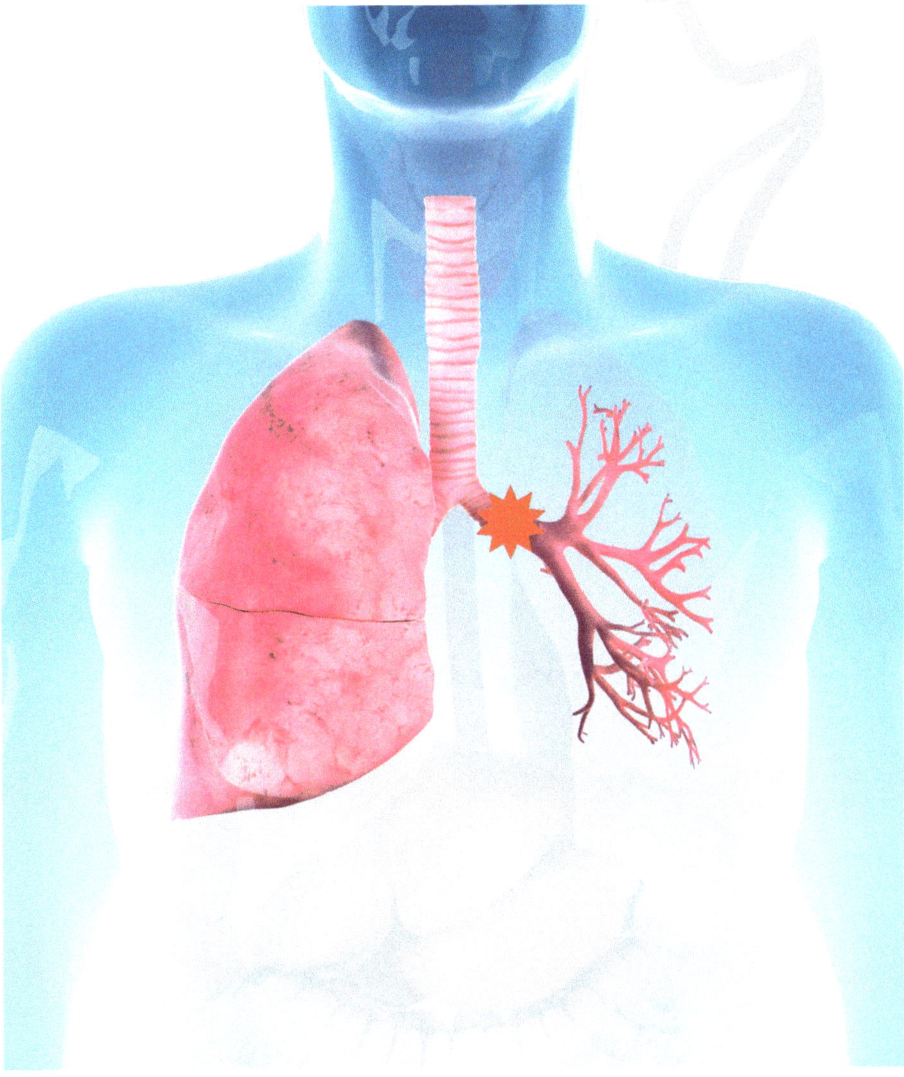

C

Cecum

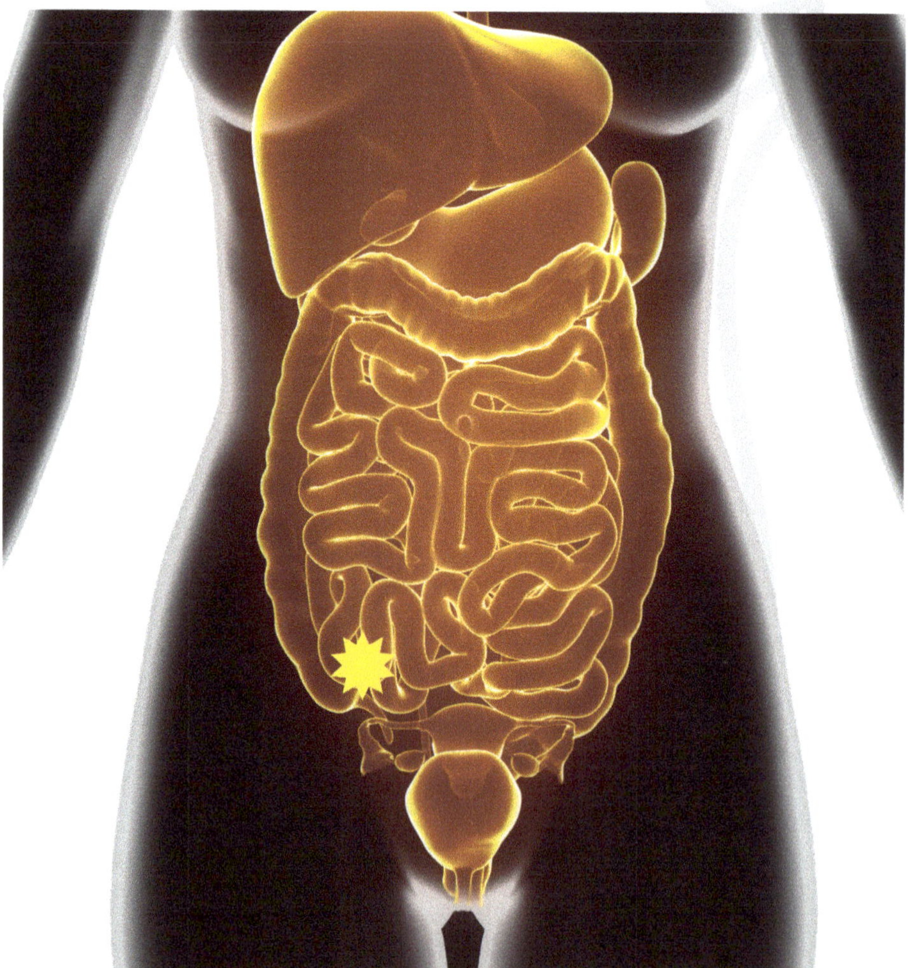

C

Cerebellum

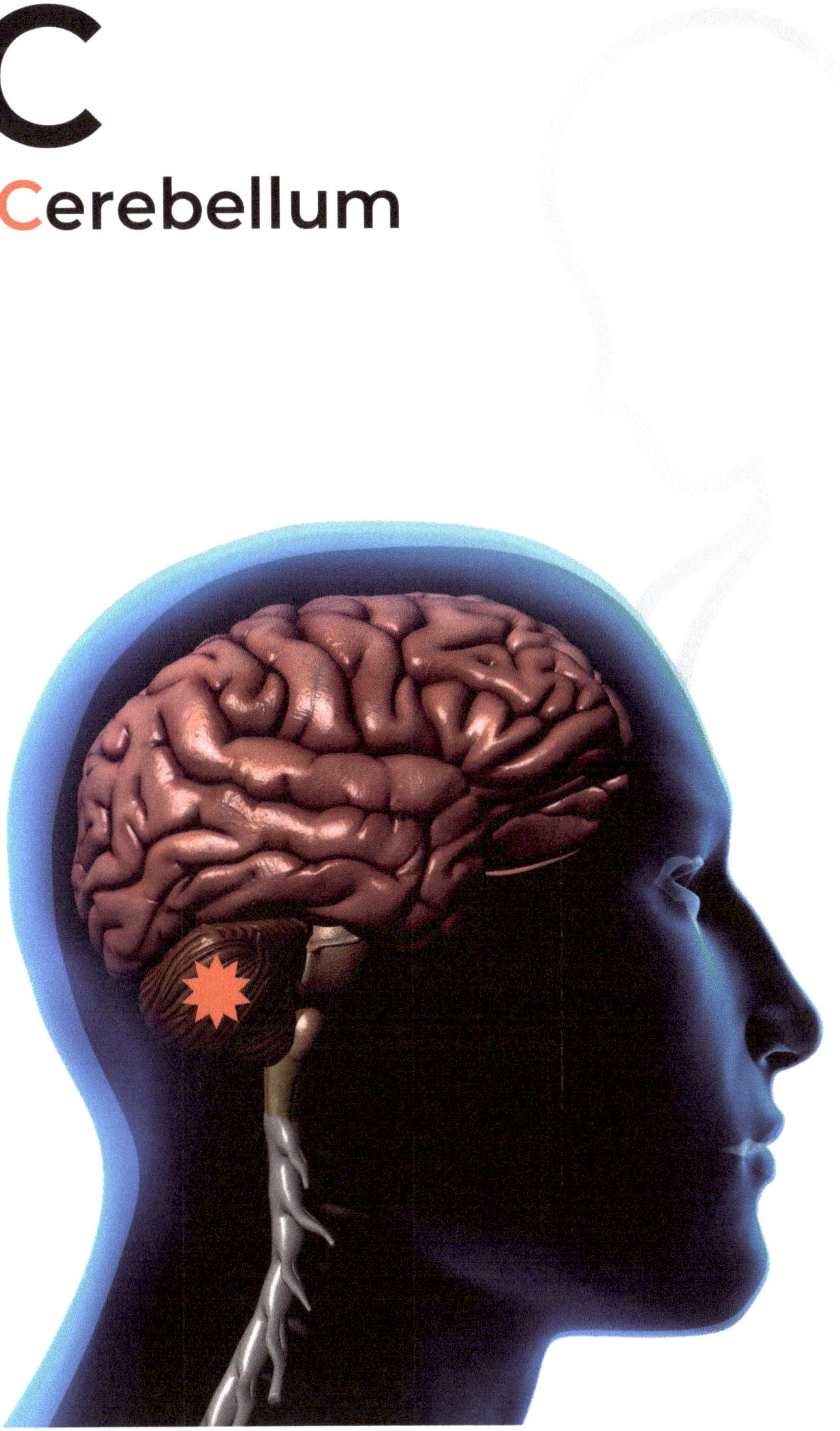

C

Cerebrum

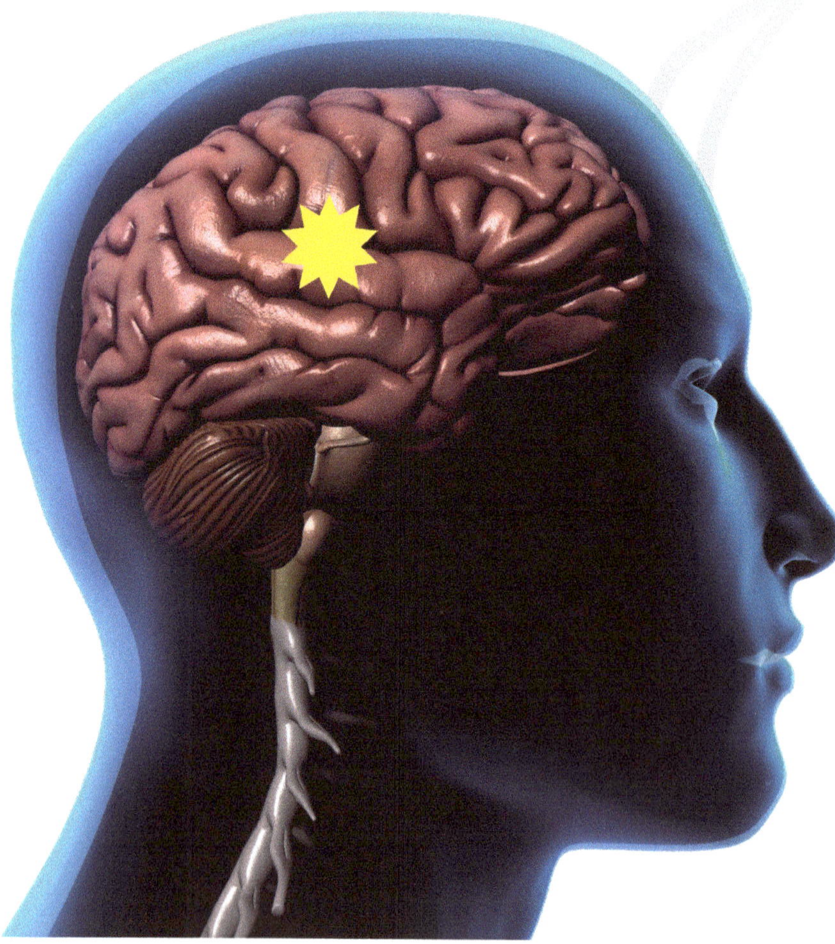

C

Common Bile Duct

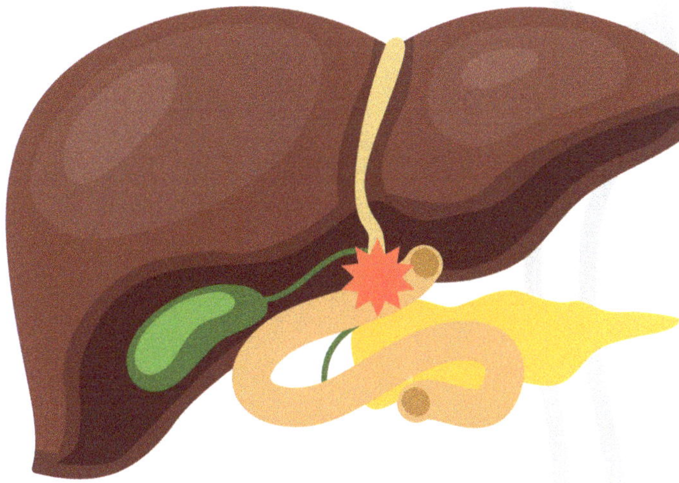

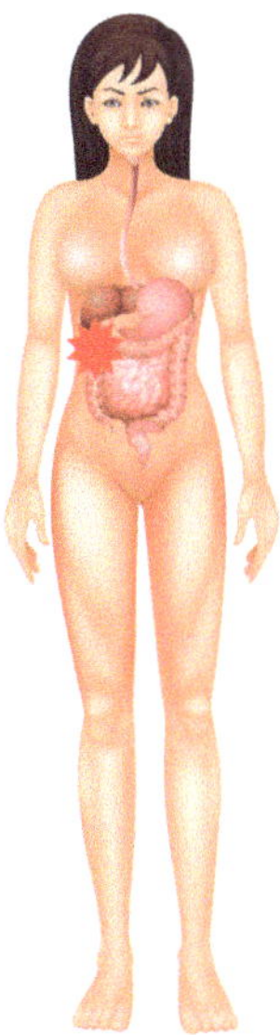

C

Conus Medullaris

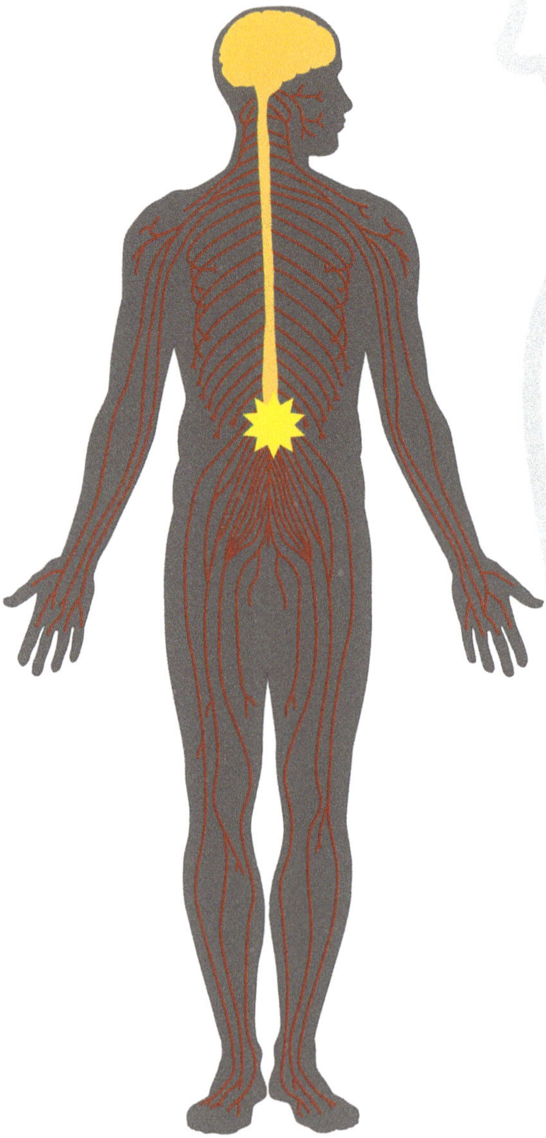

D

Deltoid (muscle)

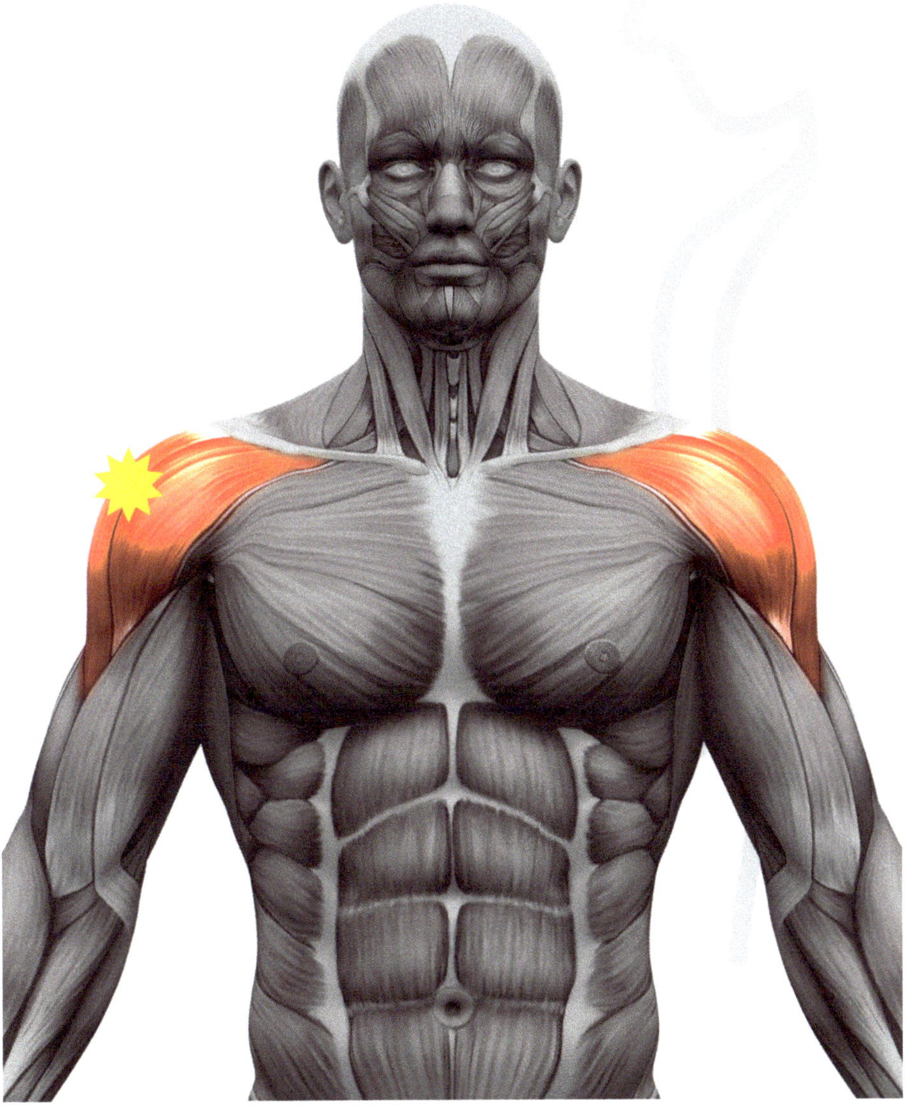

D

Descending Colon

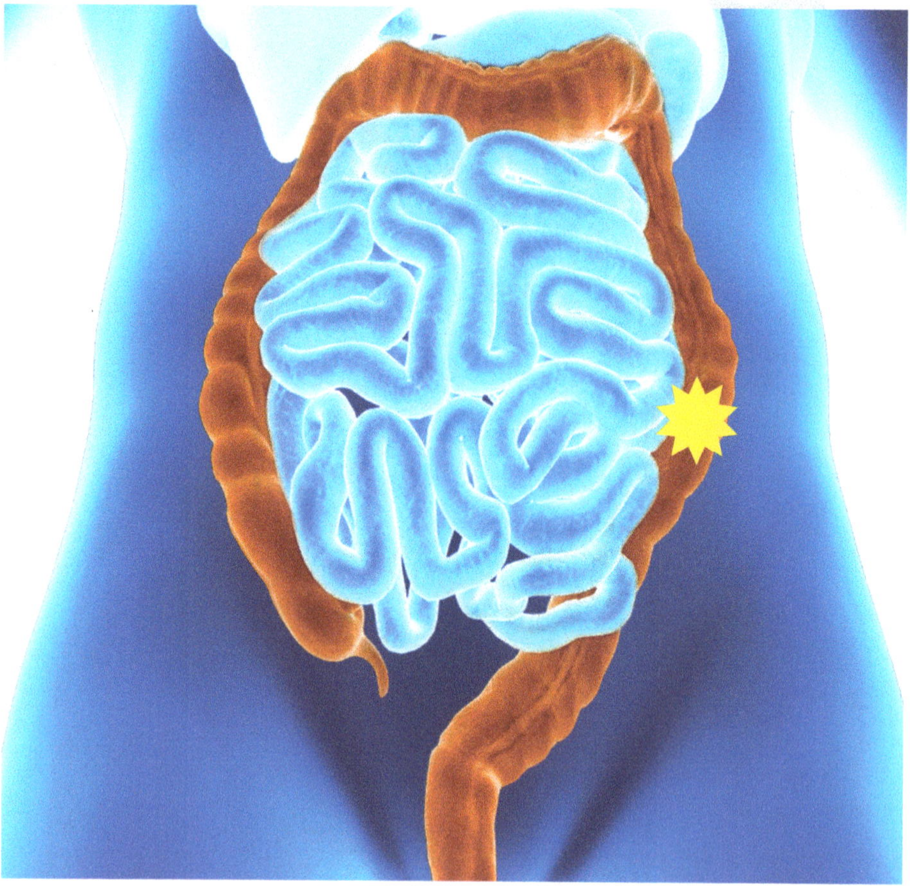

D

Diaphragm (muscle)

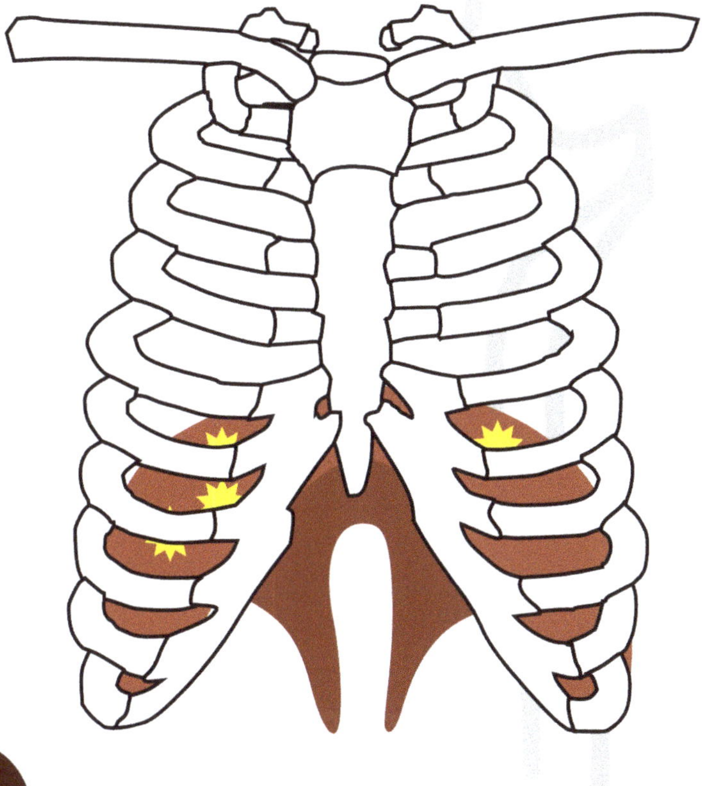

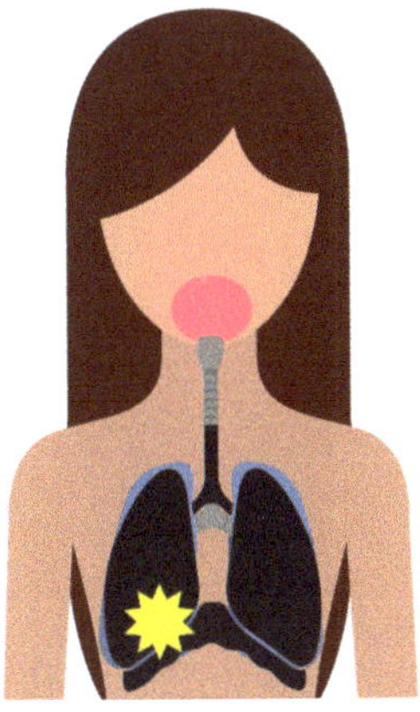

D

Duodenum

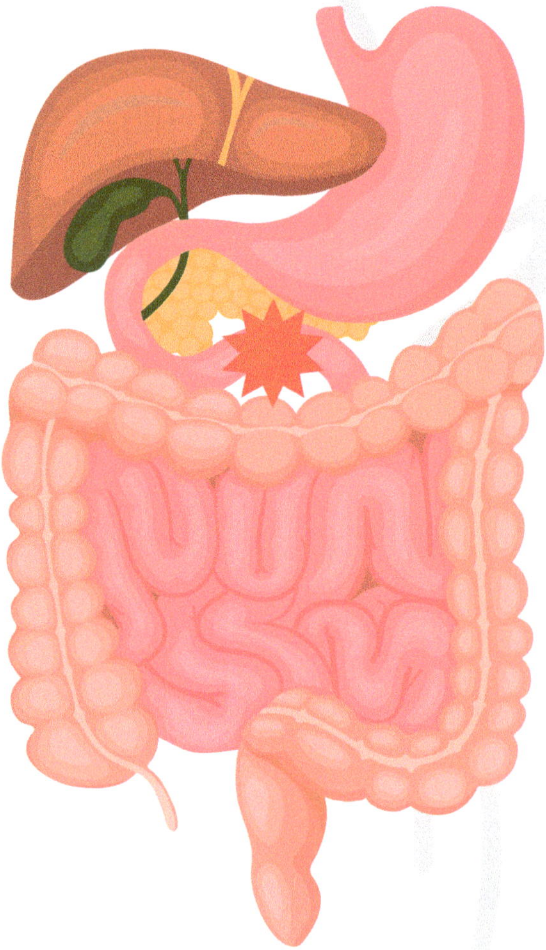

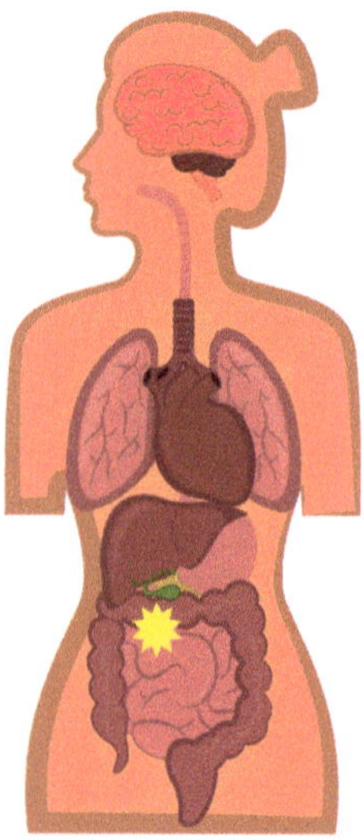

E
Epididymis

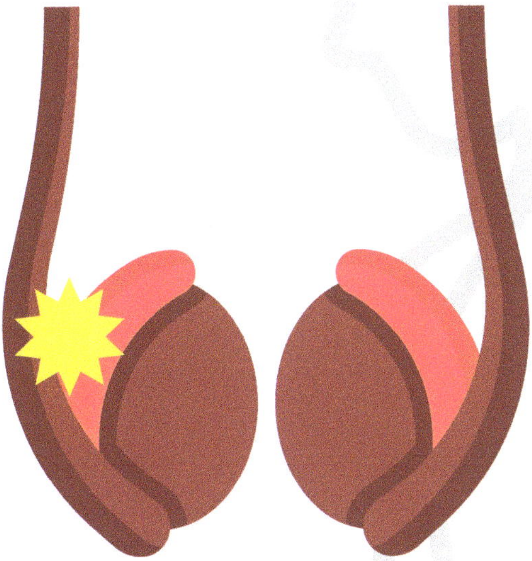

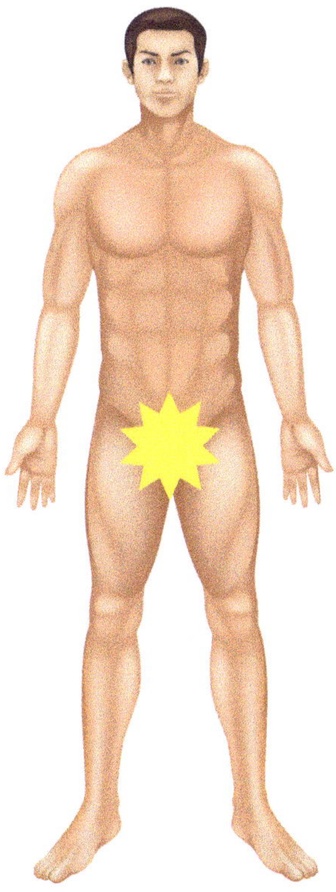

E

External Iliac Vein

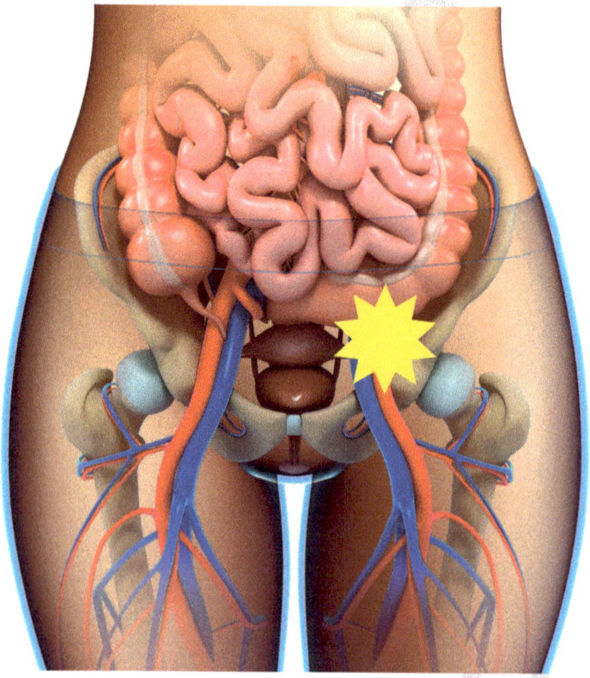

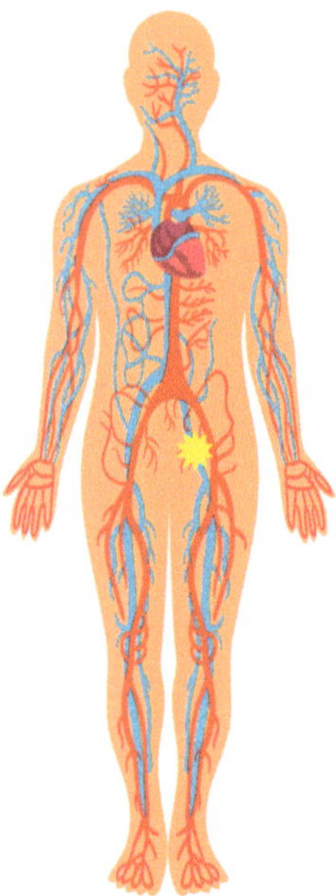

E

External Oblique (muscle)

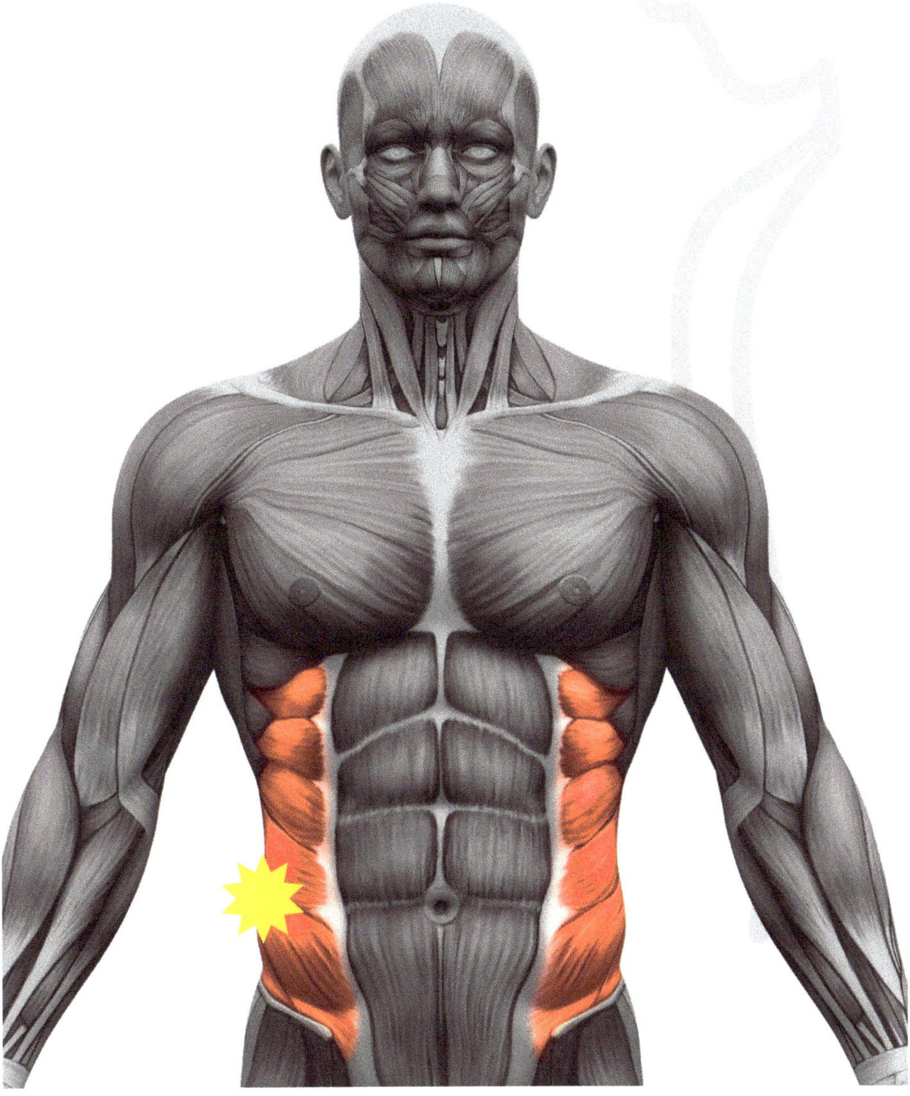

E

Eyelid

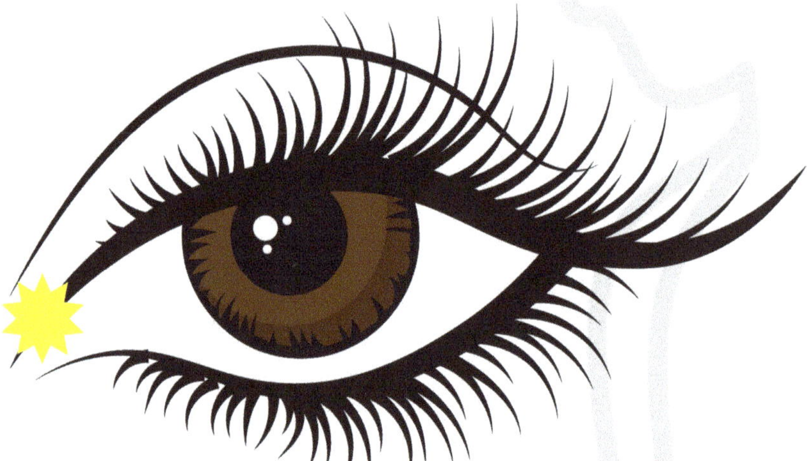

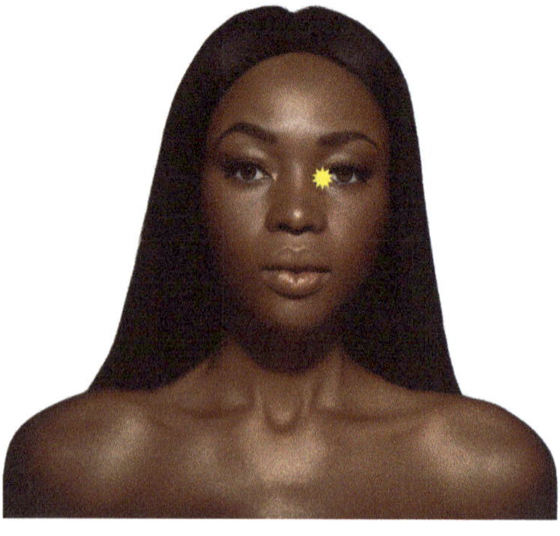

F

Falciform Ligament

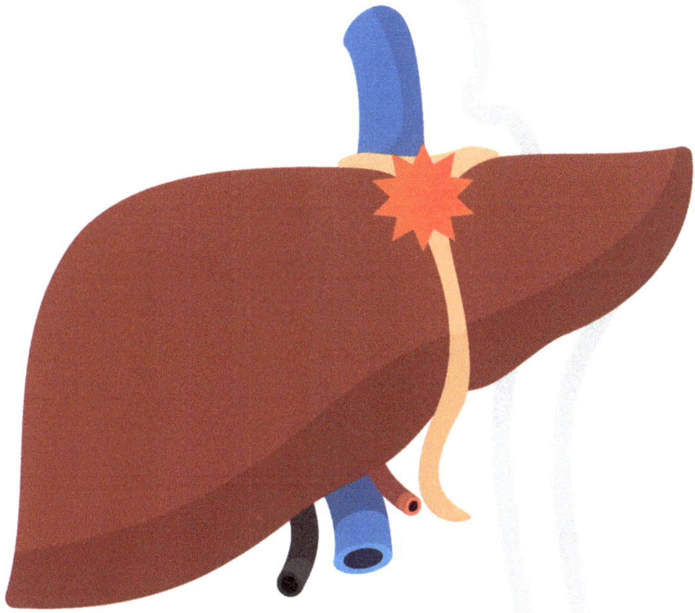

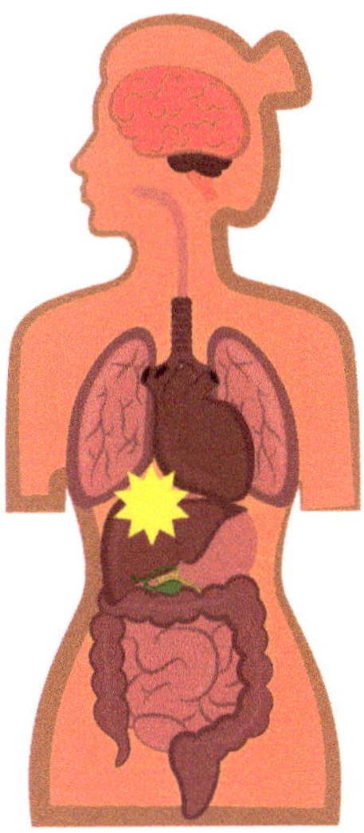

F

Femoral Nerve

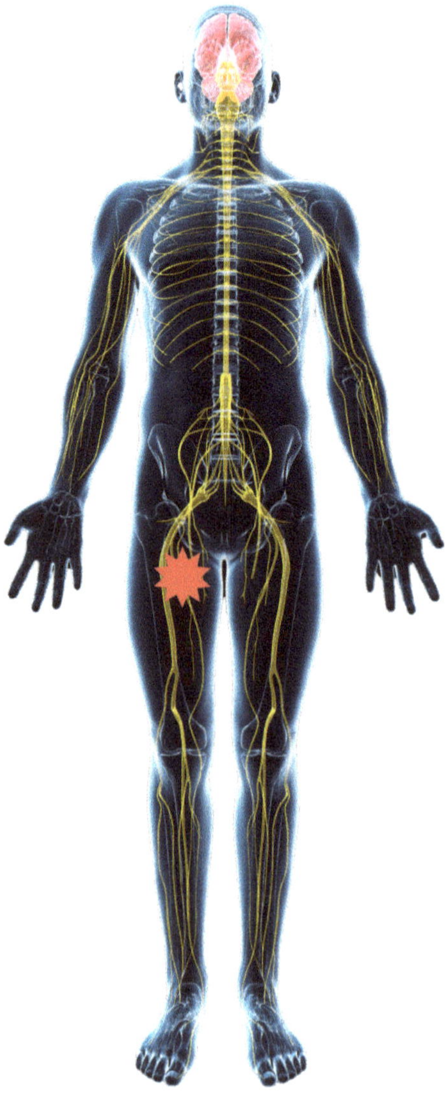

F

Femoral Vein

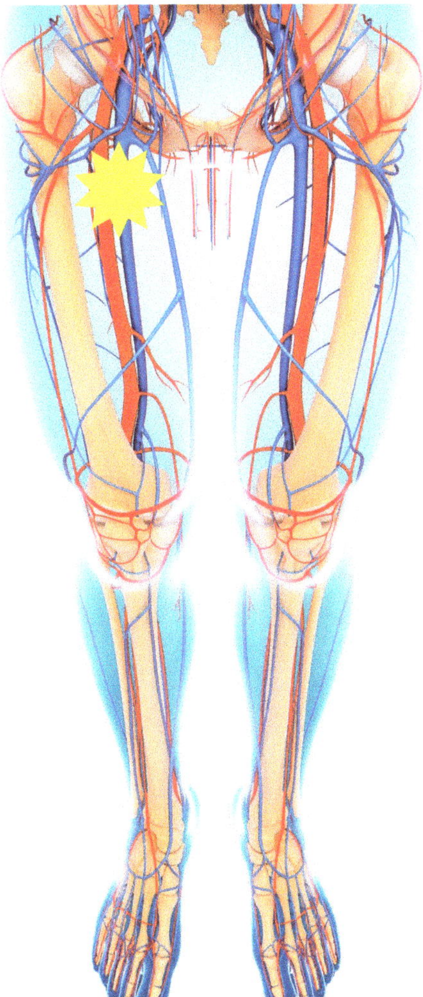

F

Femur

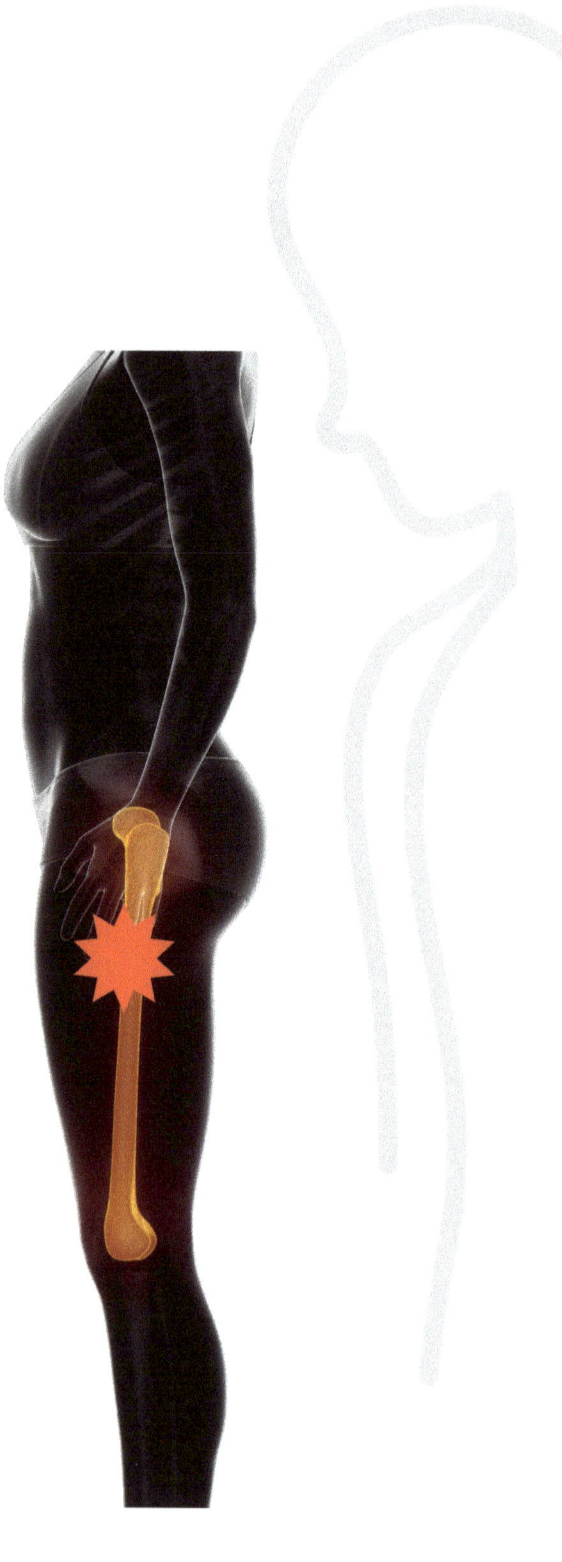

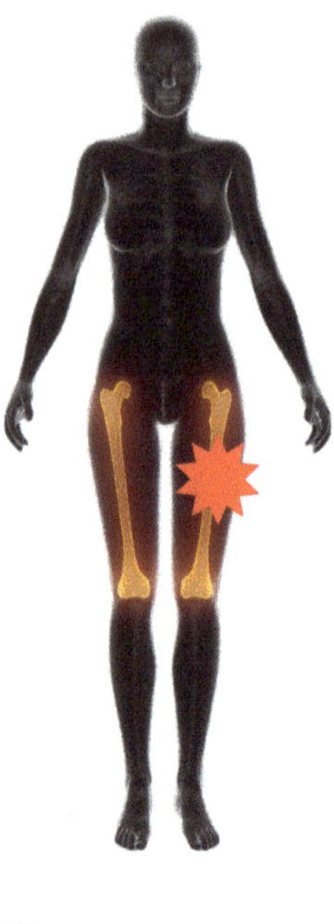

F

Fingertip

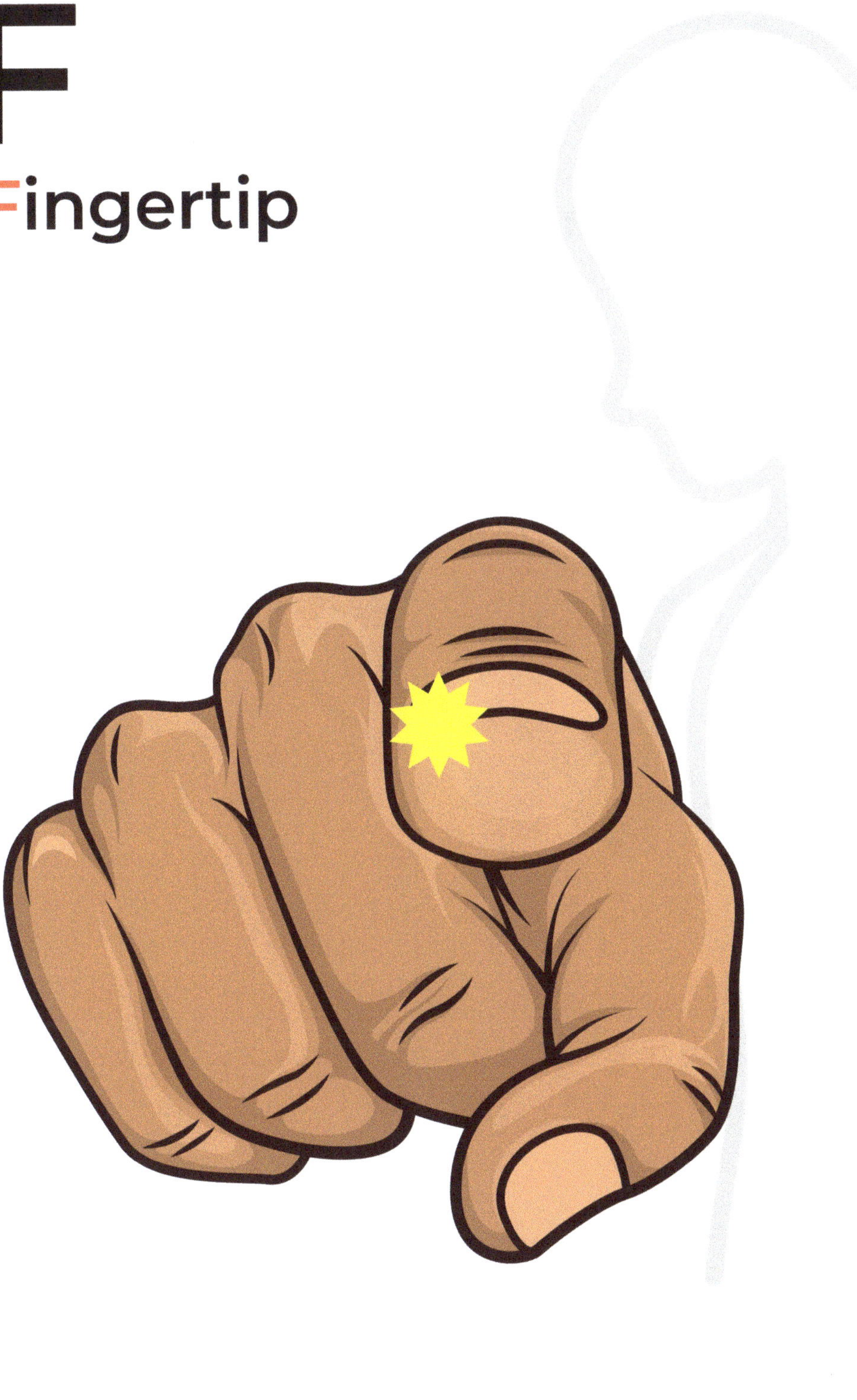

G

Gallbladder

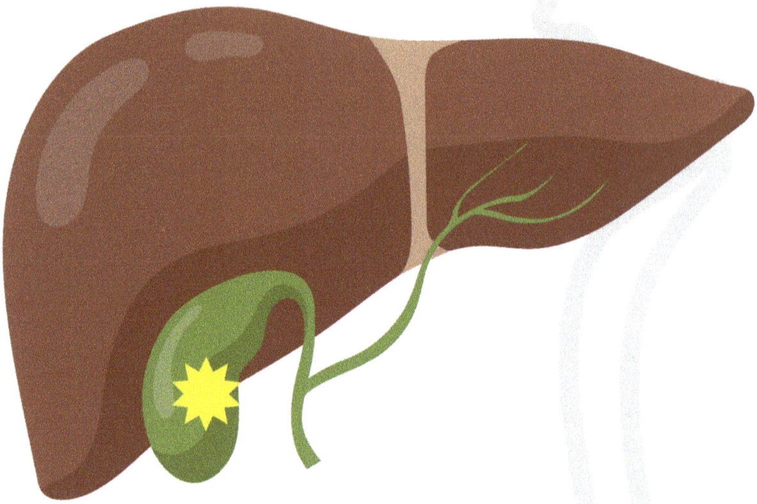

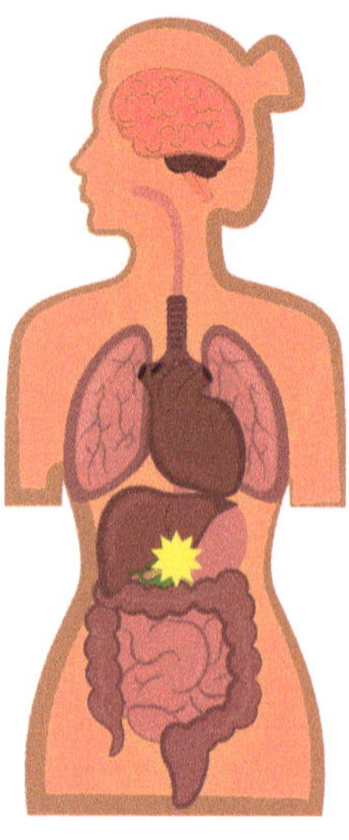

G

Gastrocnemius (muscle)

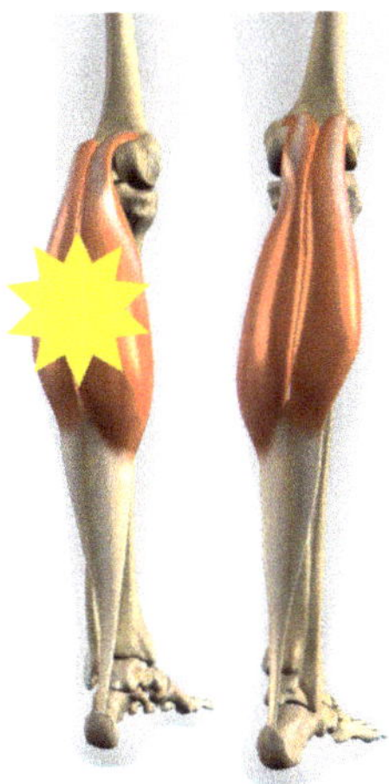

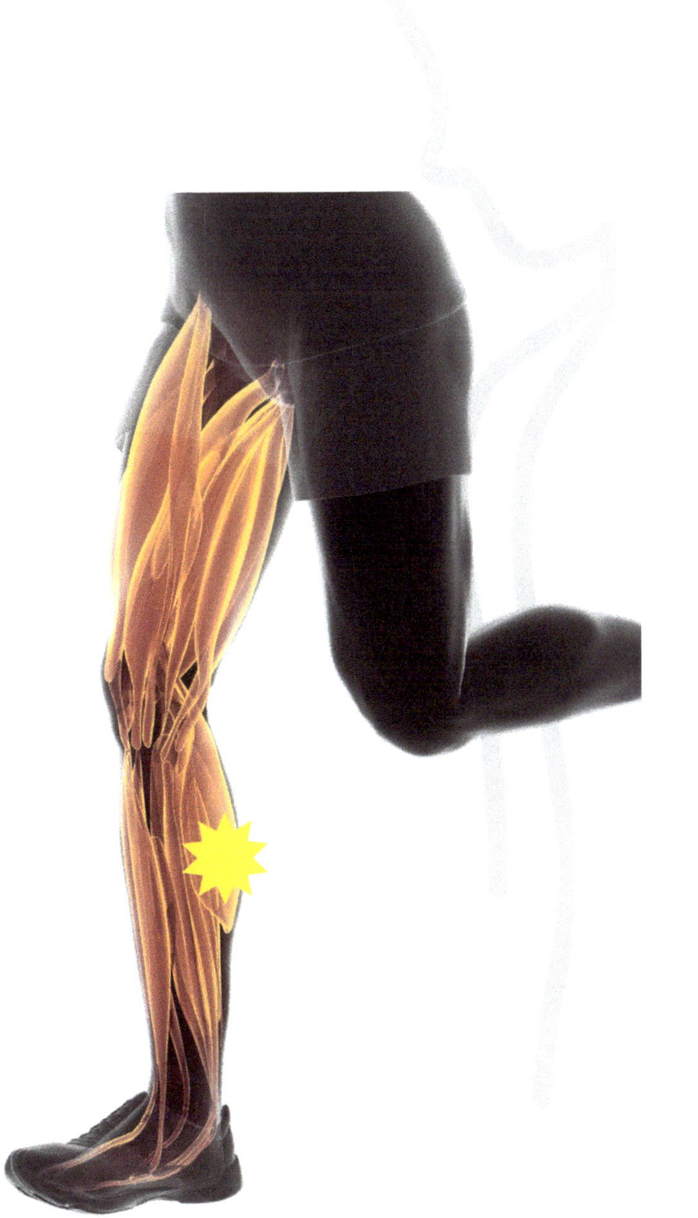

G

Gluteus Maximus
Gluteus Medius
(muscles)

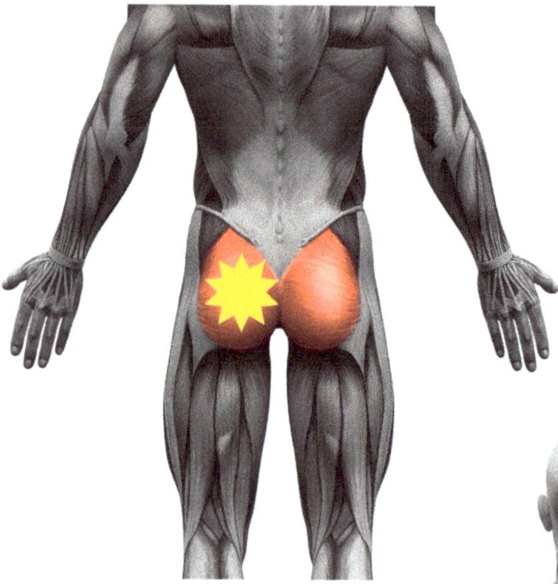

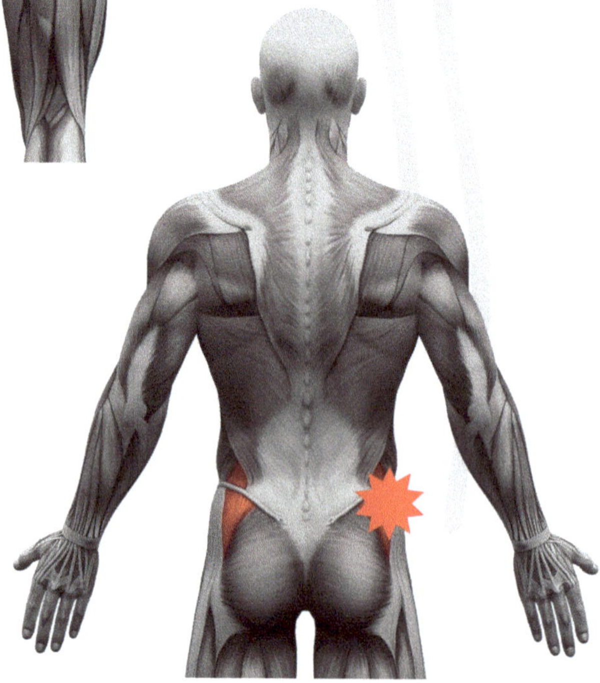

G
Groin

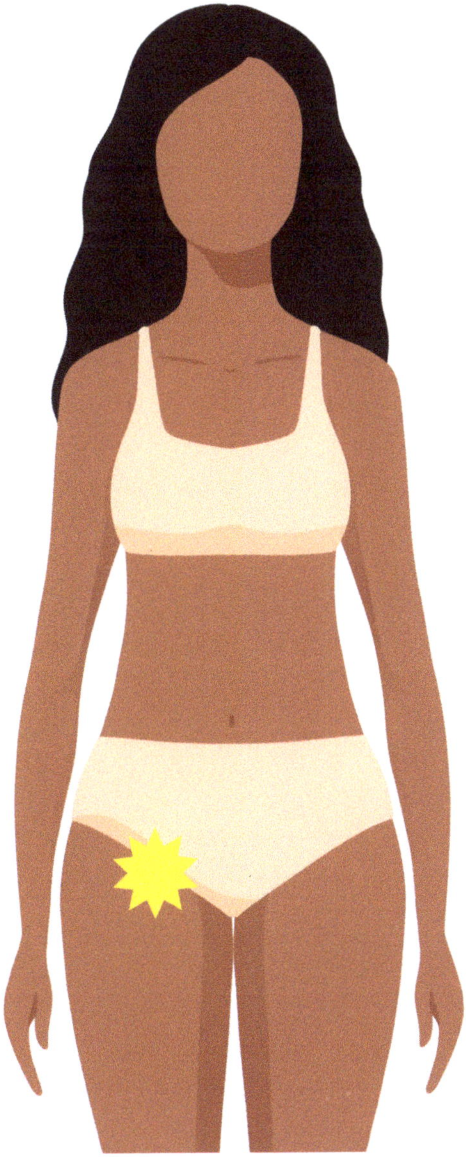

H

Heart

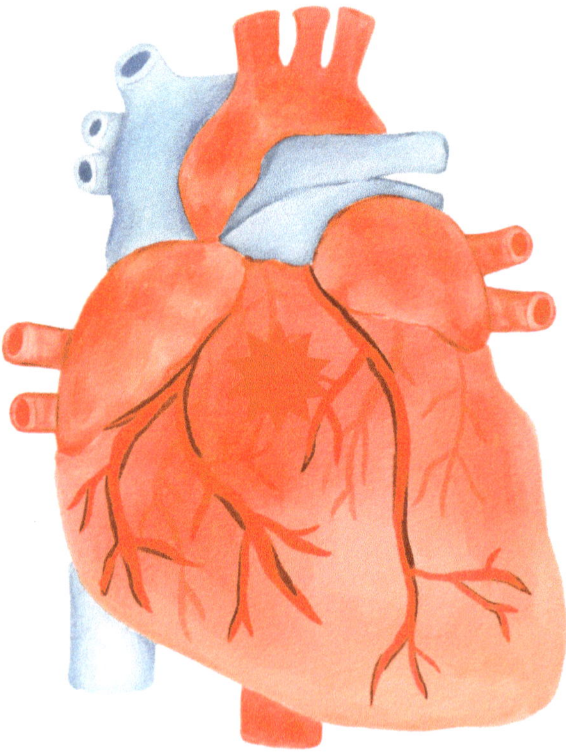

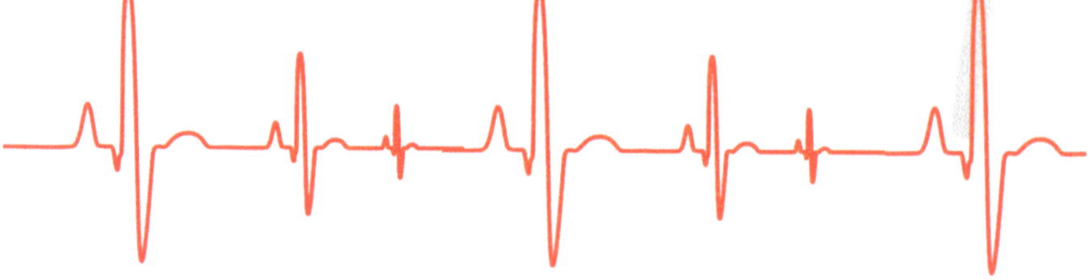

I

Ileum

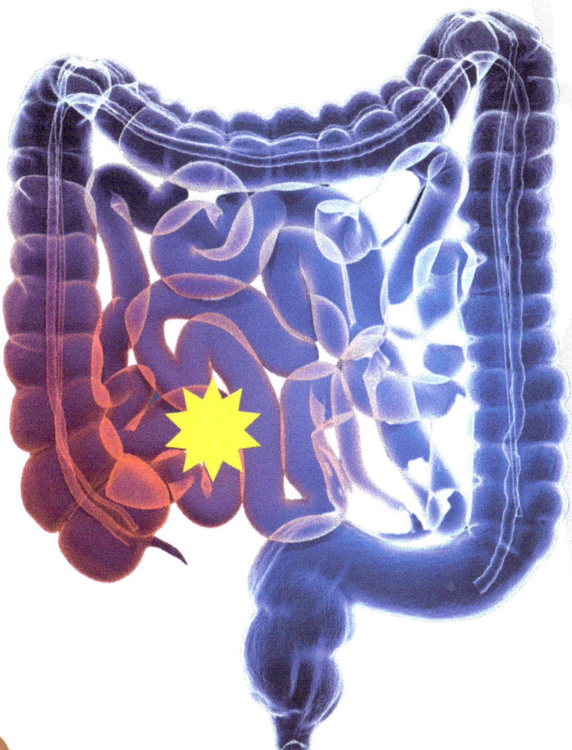

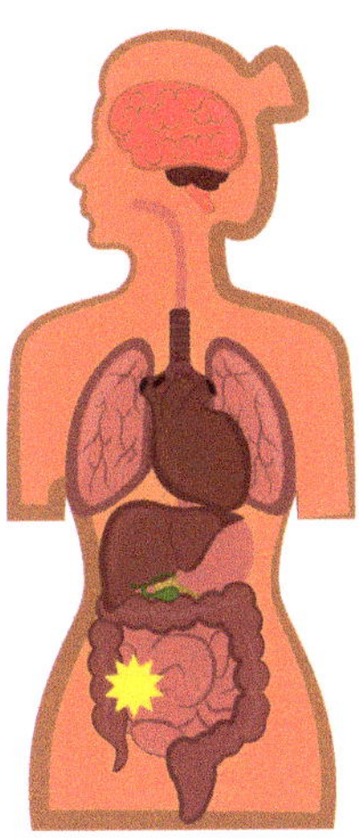

I

Ileocecal Valve

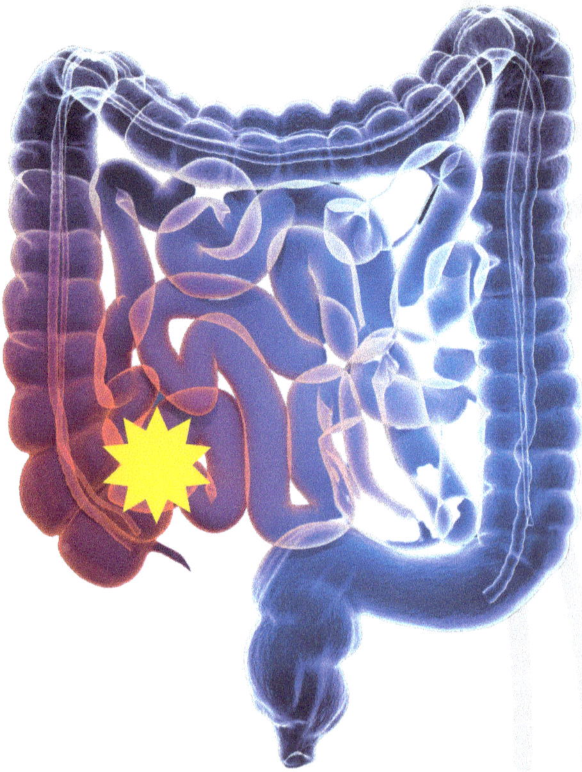

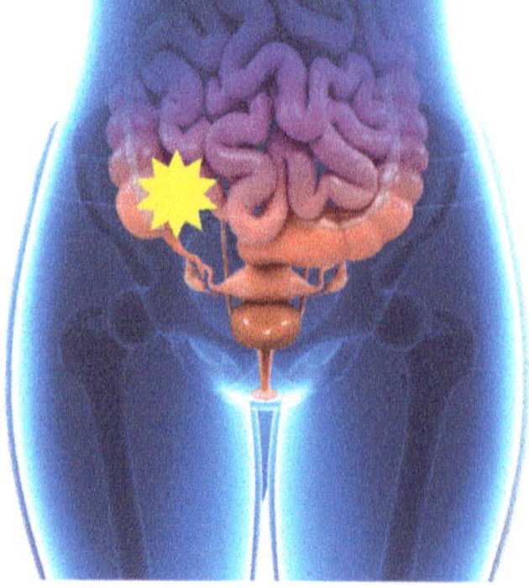

I

Ilioinguinal Nerve

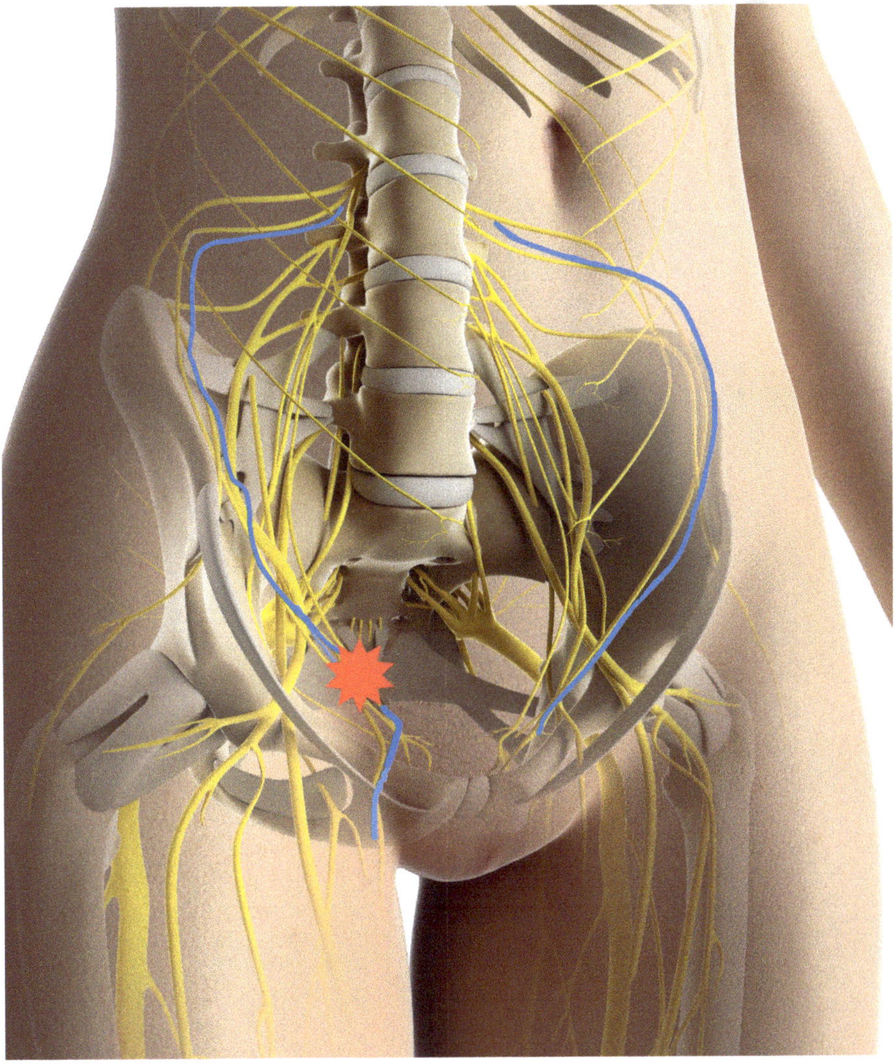

I

Inferior Vena Cava
(Abdominal)

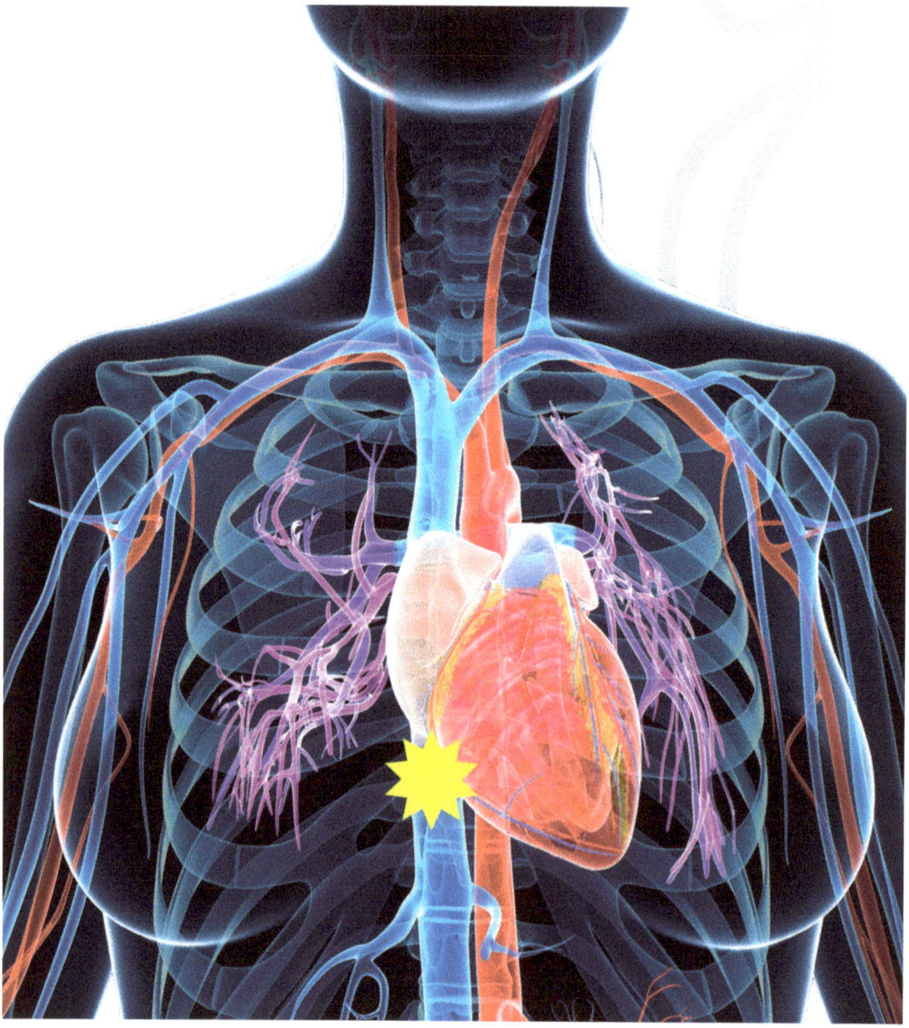

I

Inguinal Ligament and Canal

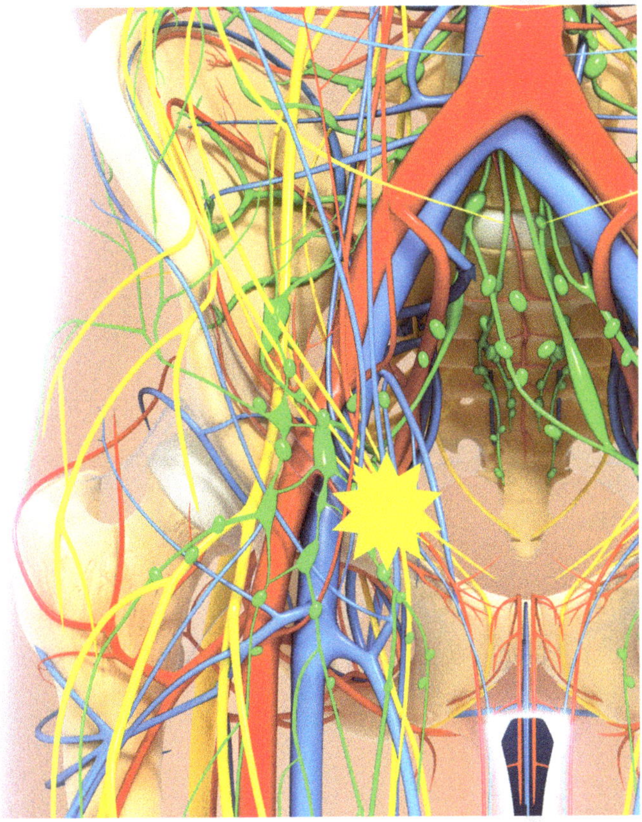

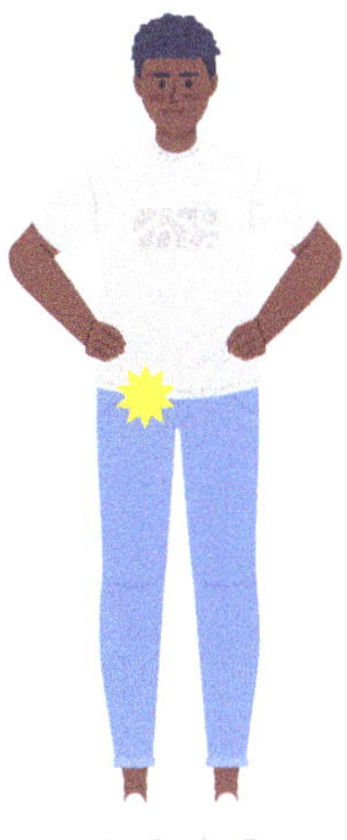

I

Ischiorectal Fossa

(not pictured)

J

Jejunum

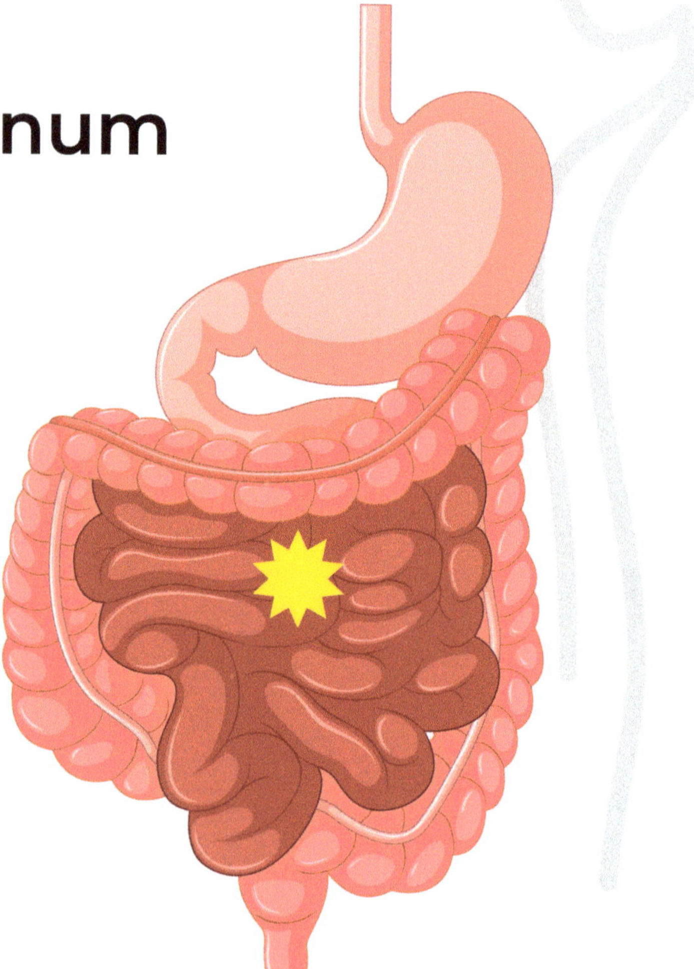

K

Kidney

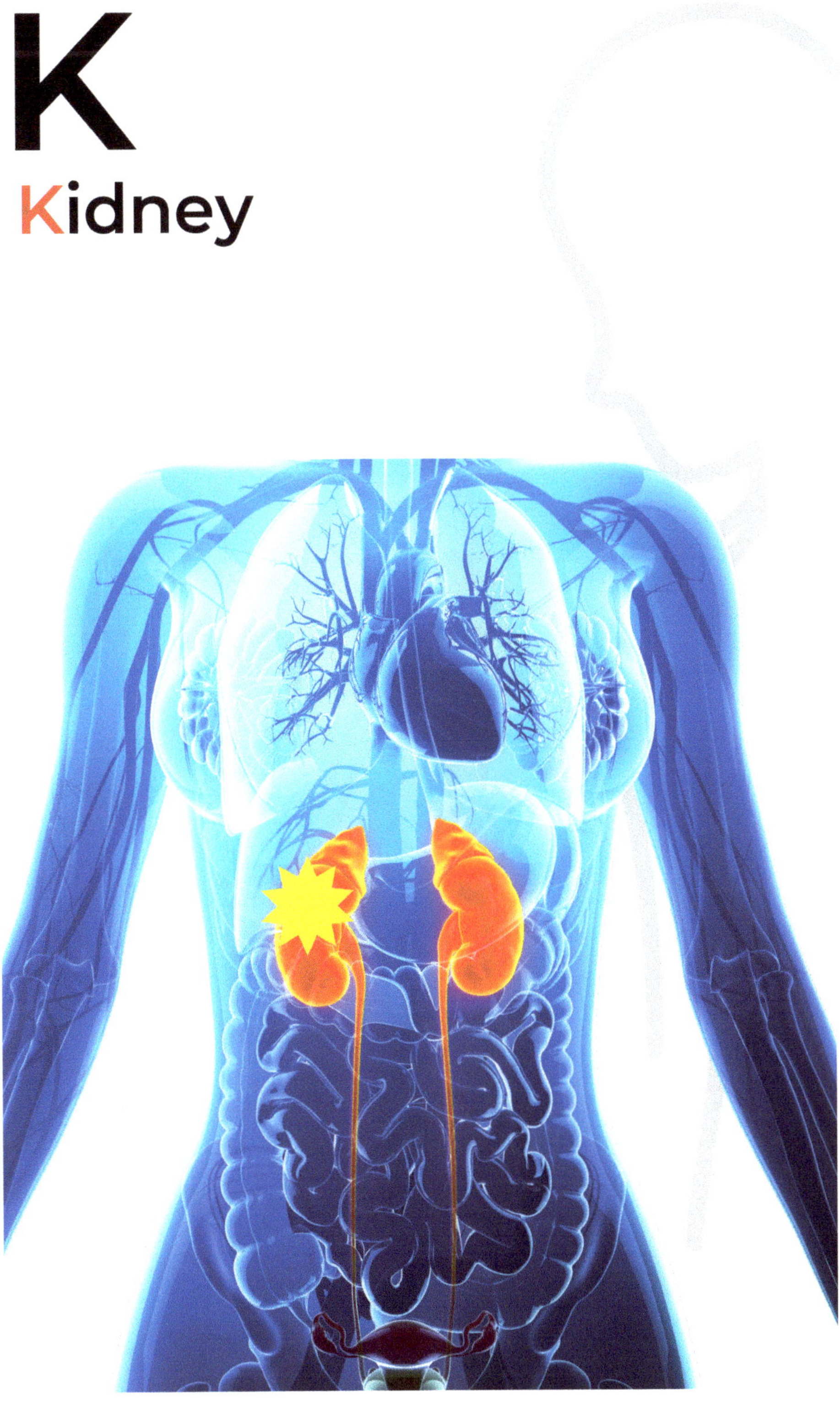

K

Knee

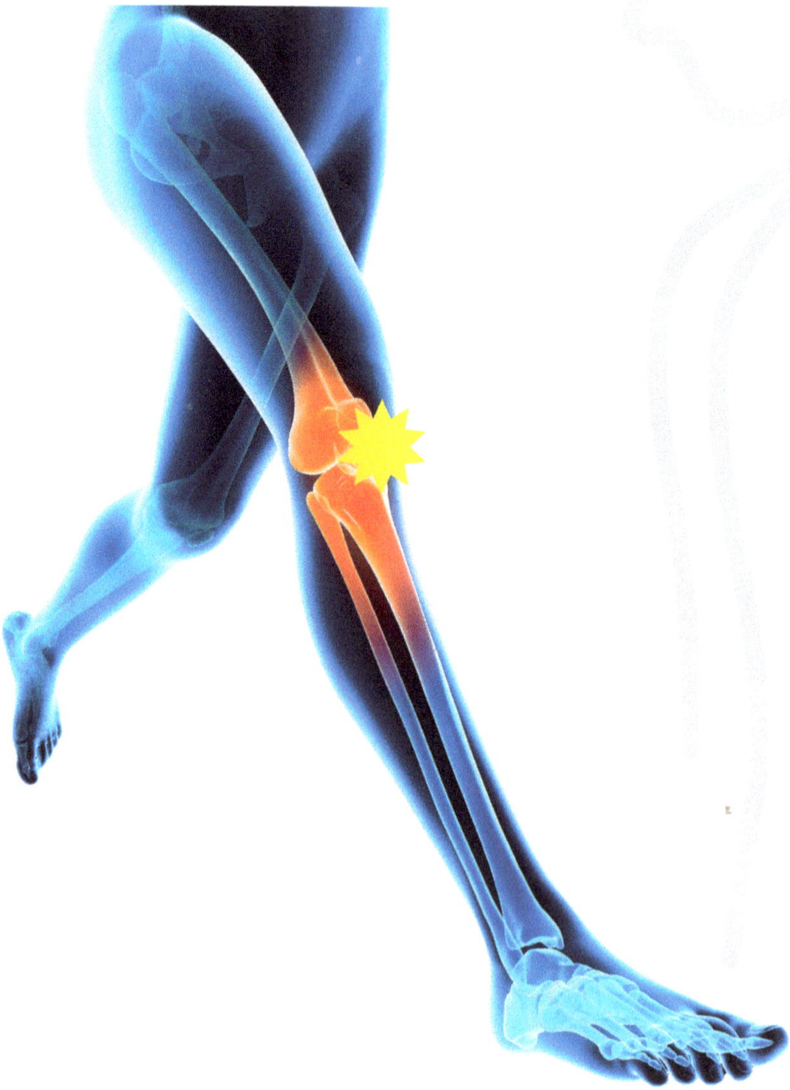

L

Lip

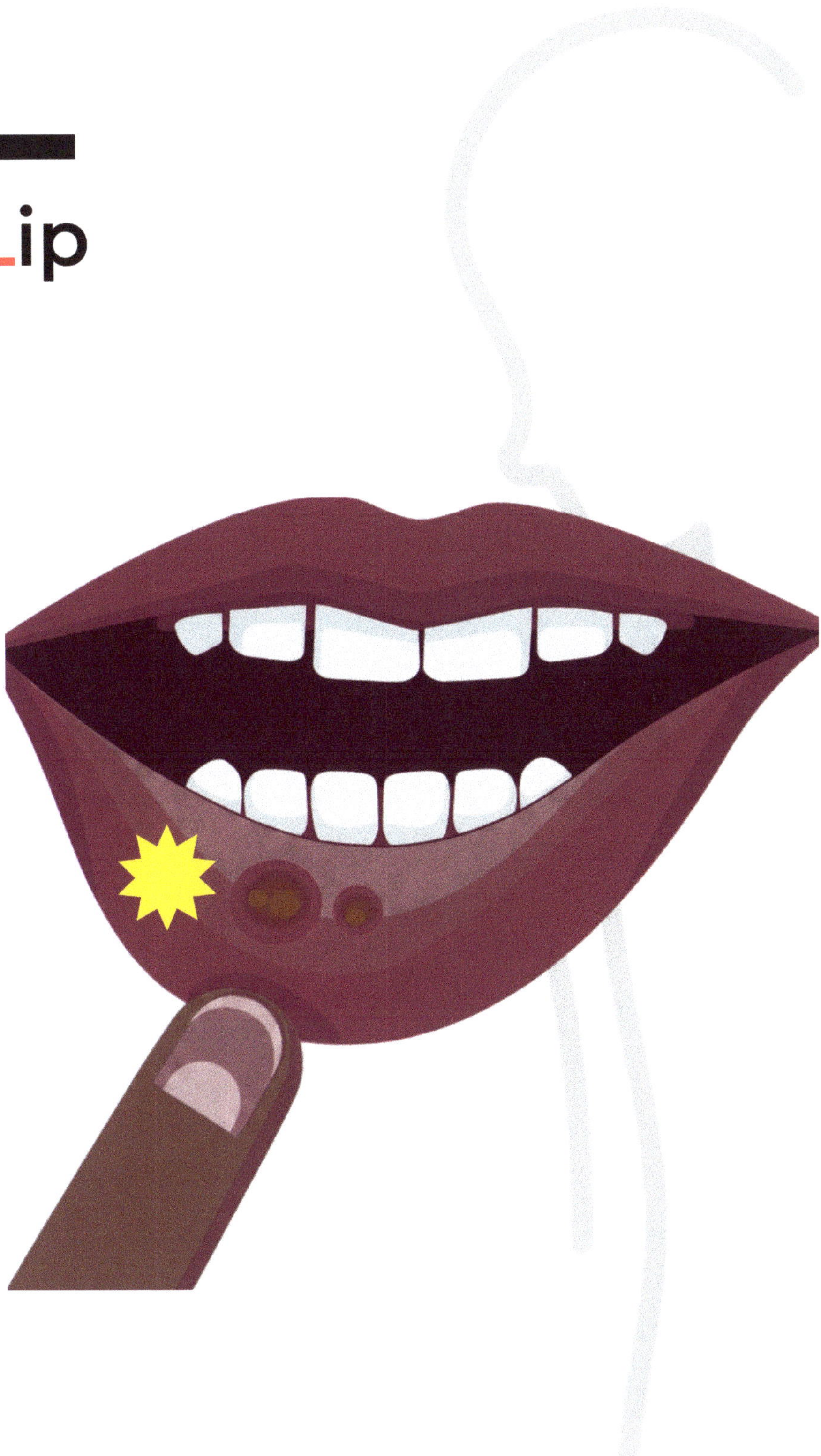

L
Liver

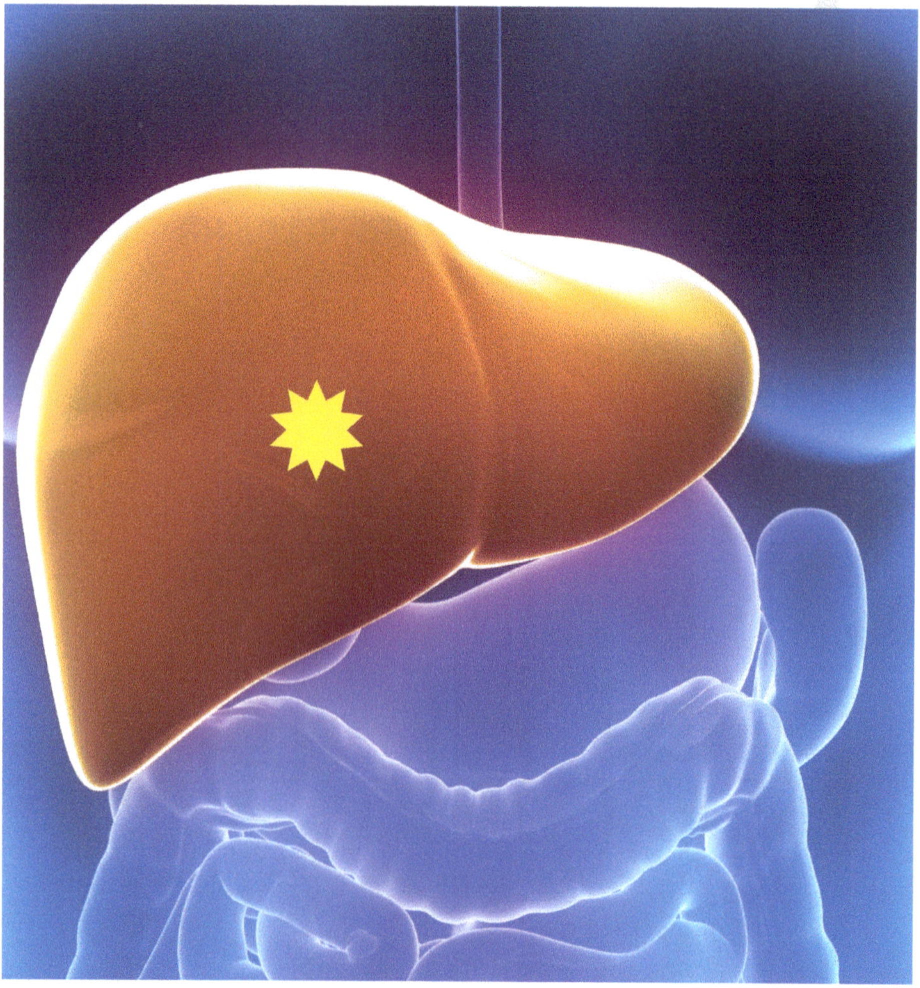

L

Lymph Nodes

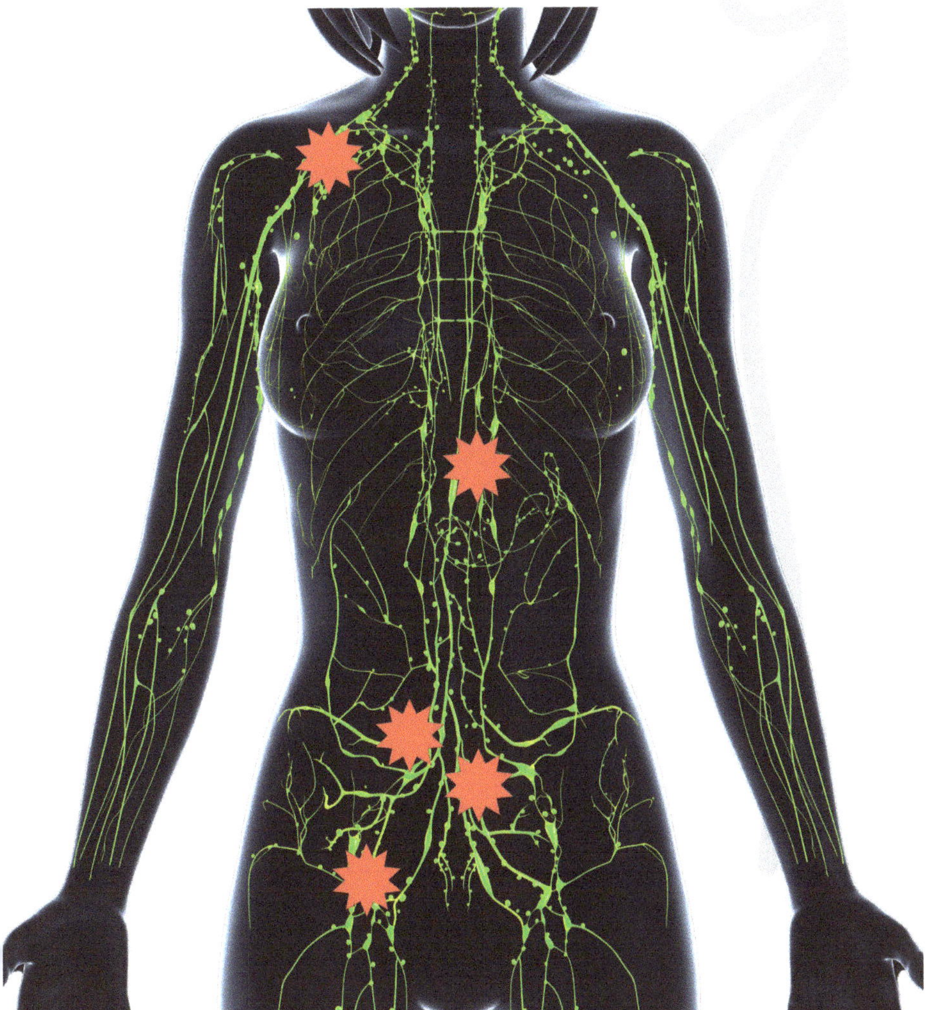

M

Mandible

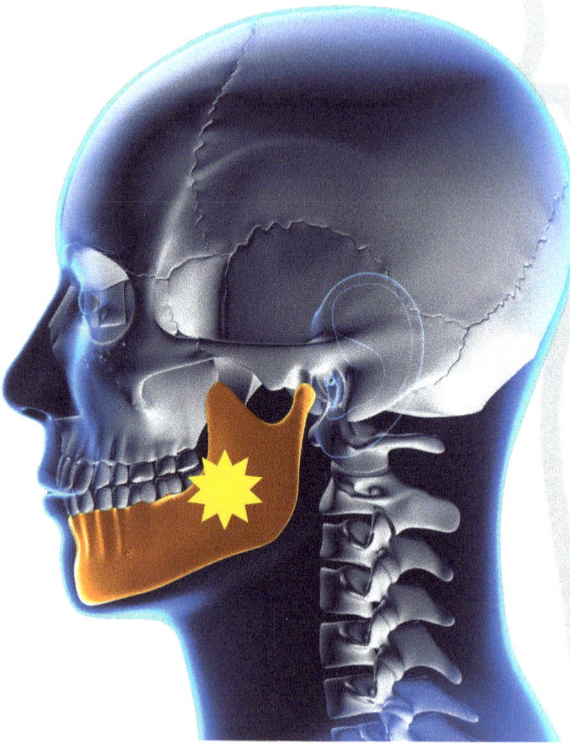

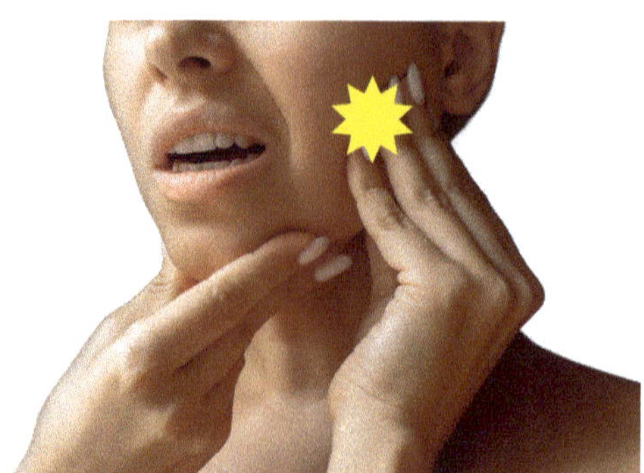

M

Mediastinum

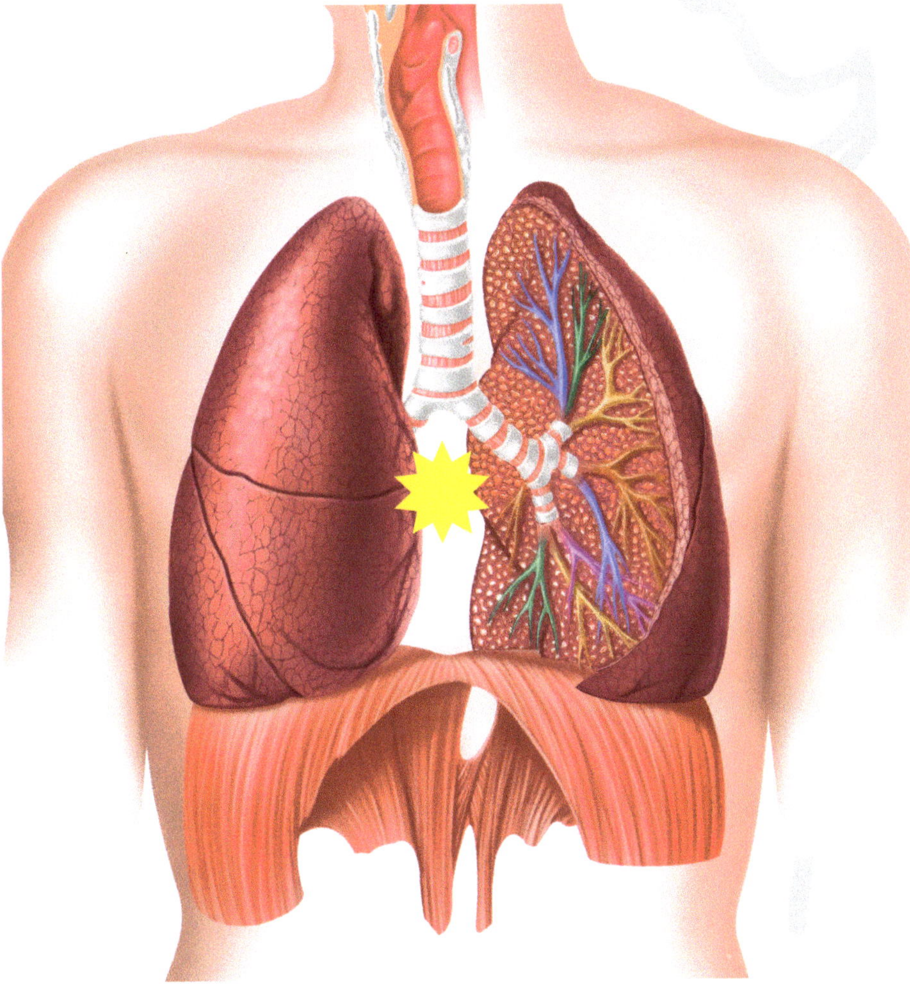

M

Mesentery

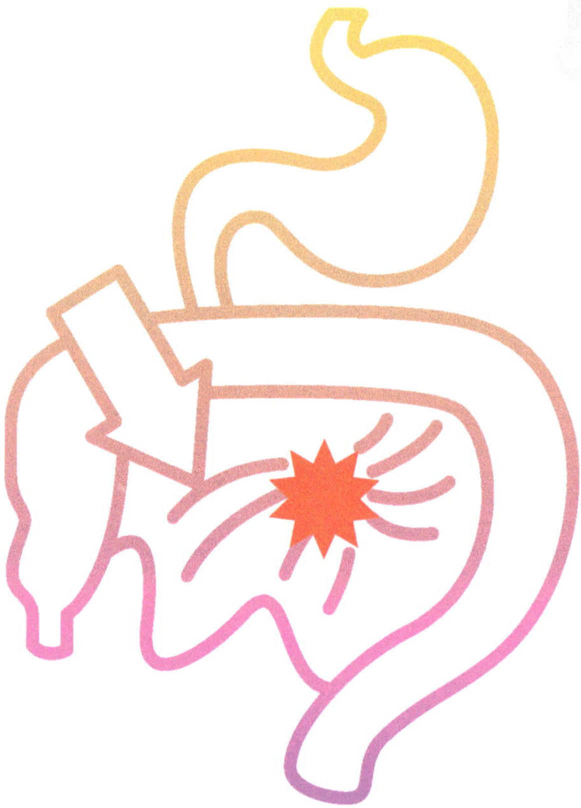

The mesentery is a continuous set of tissues located in your abdomen. It attaches your intestines to the wall of your abdomen and holds them in place.

healthline.com

N
Nerve Root

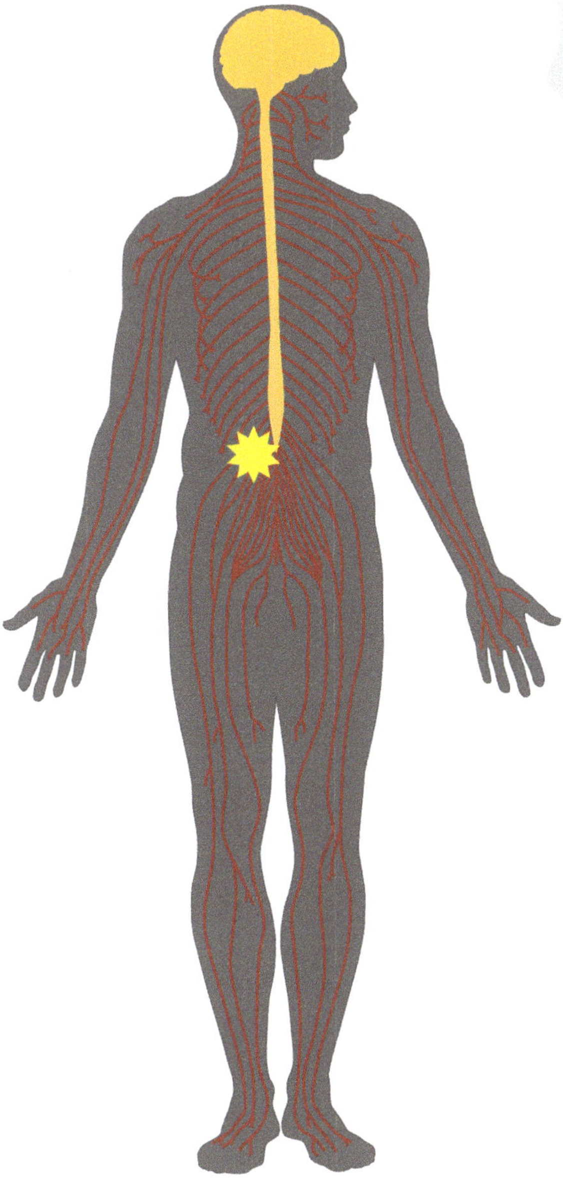

N

Nose (Nasal Mucosa)

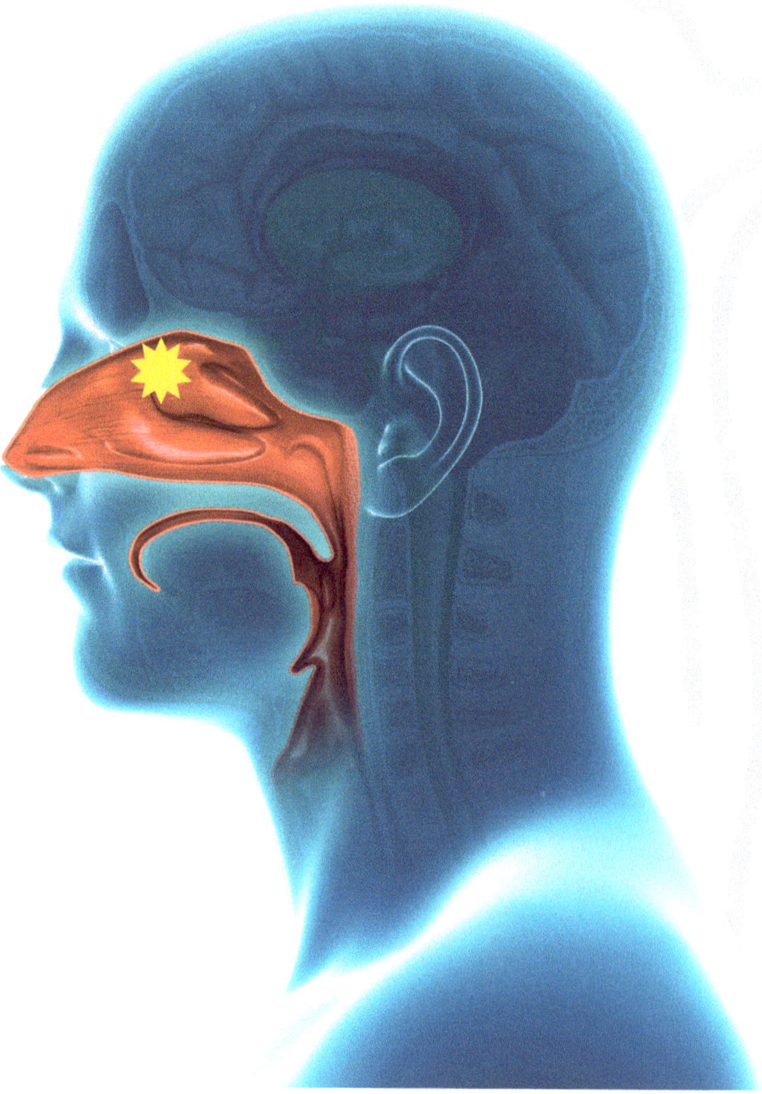

O

Obturator Internus (muscle)

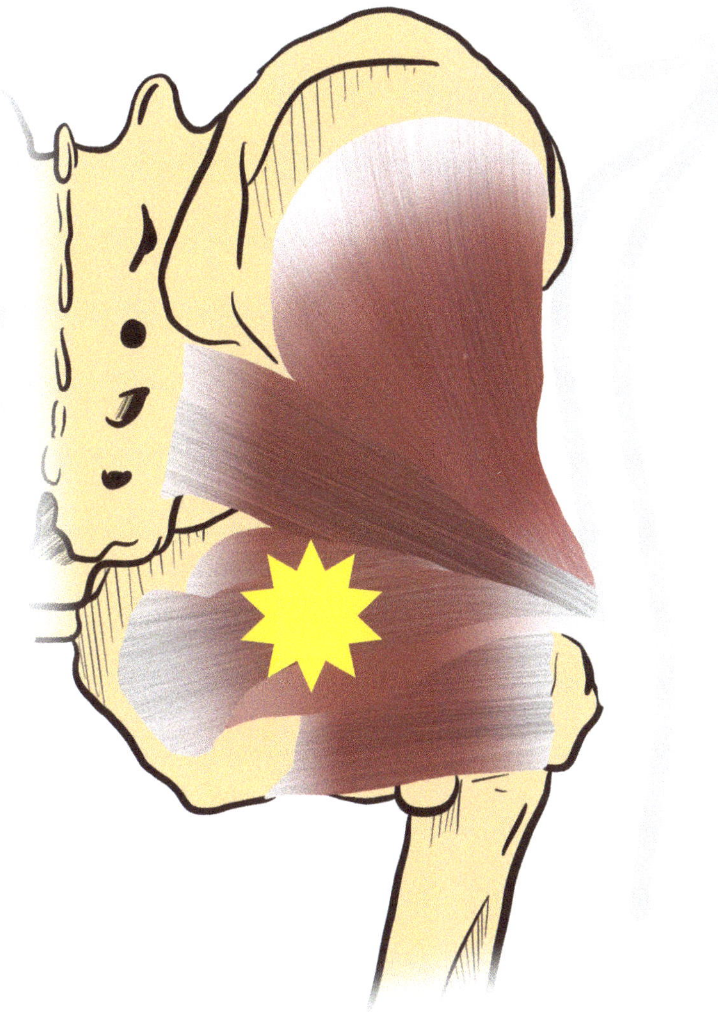

O

Obturator Nerve

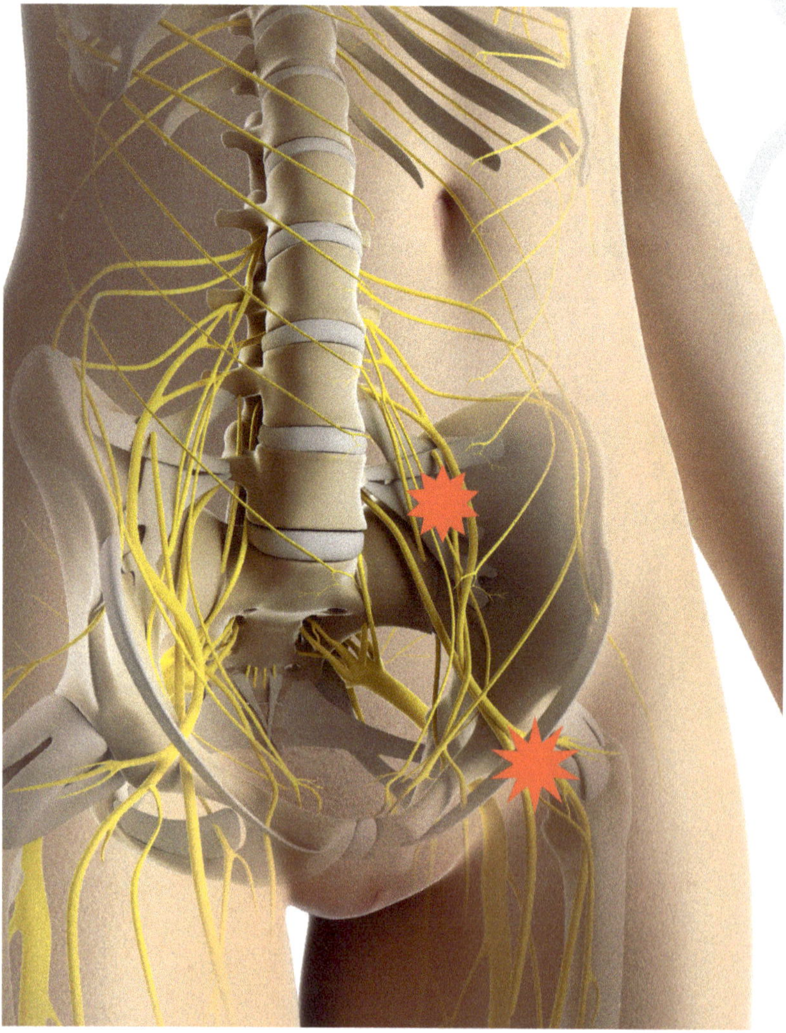

O

Omentum

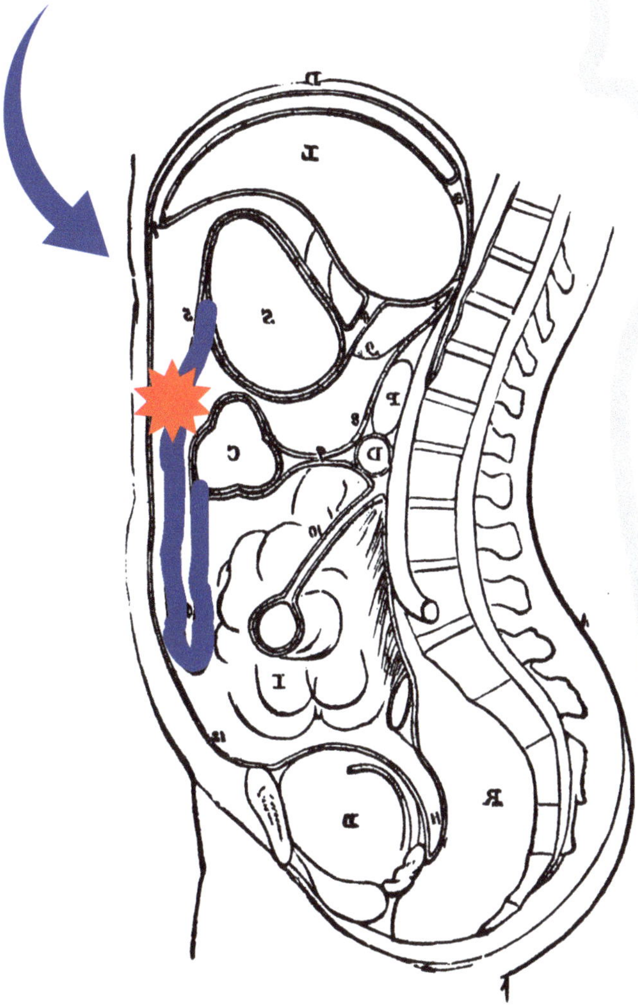

A fold of peritoneum extending from the stomach to adjacent abdominal organs.
thefreedictionary.com

P

Pancreas

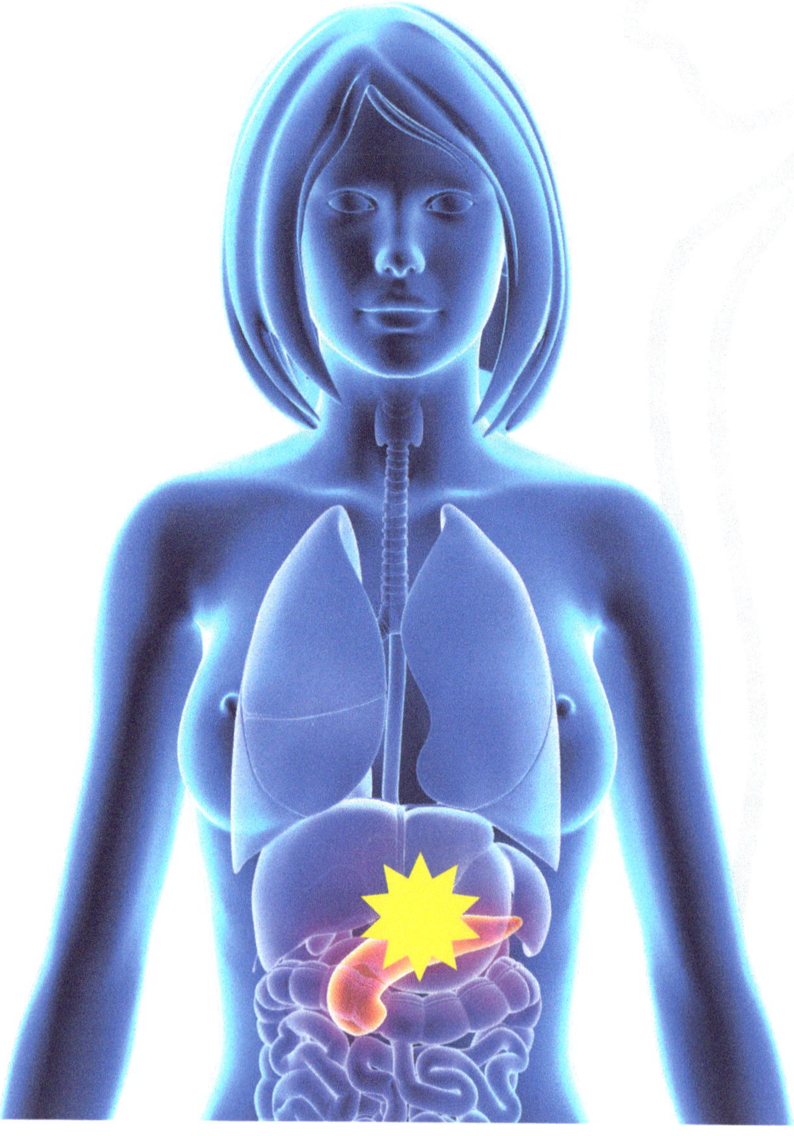

P

Parietal Pleura

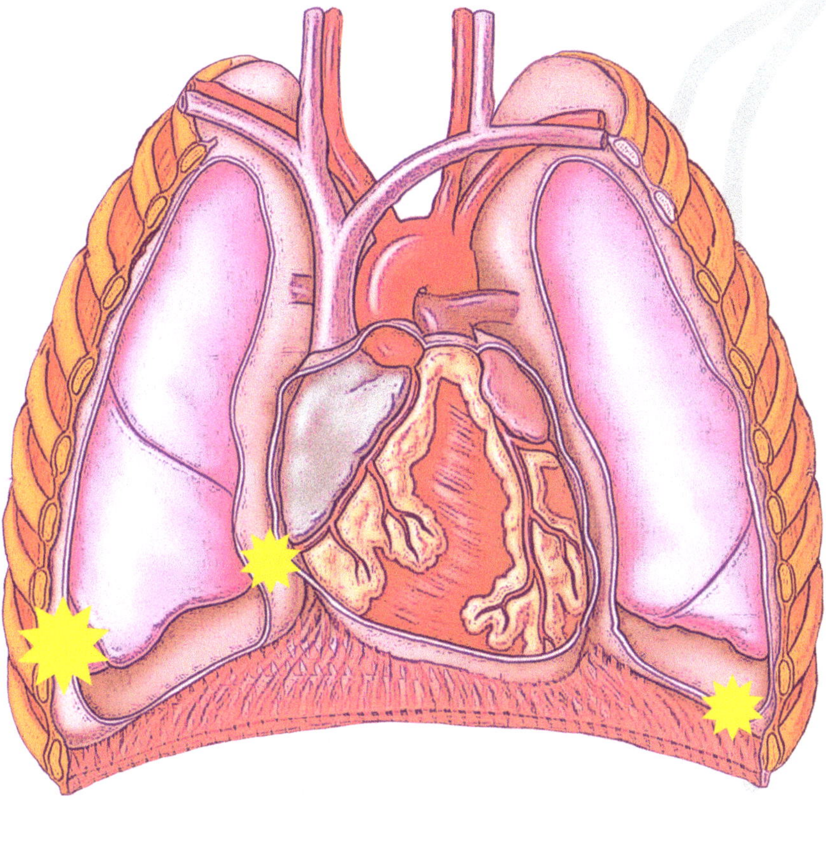

P
Perianal

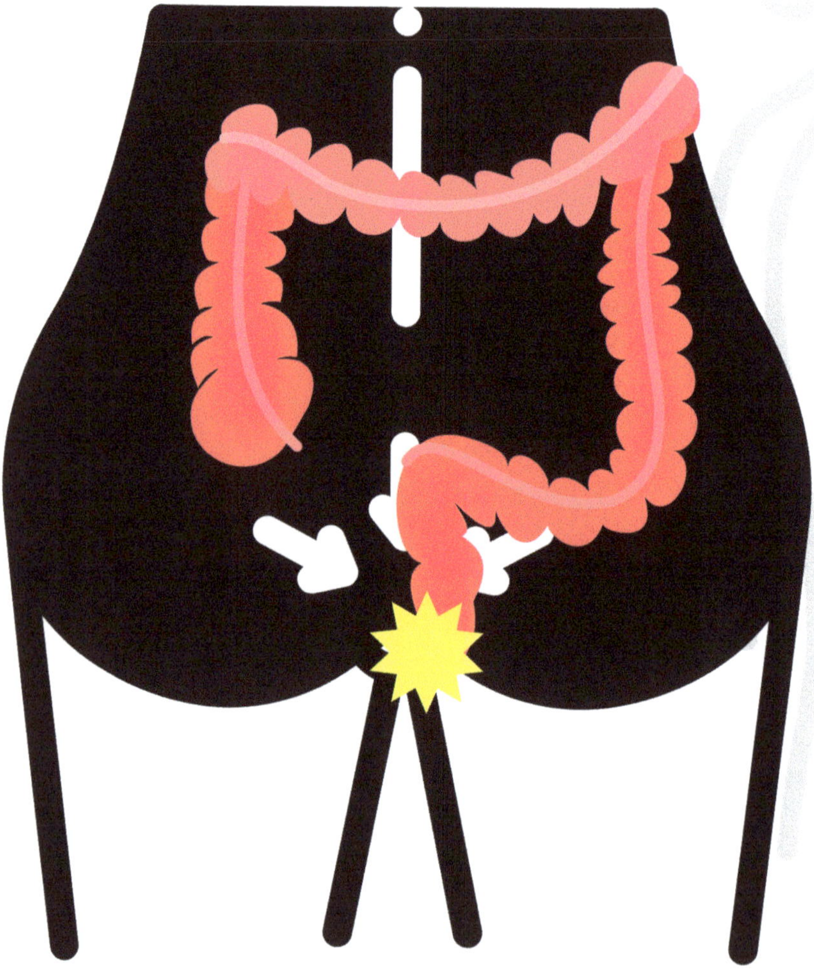

P

Pericardium

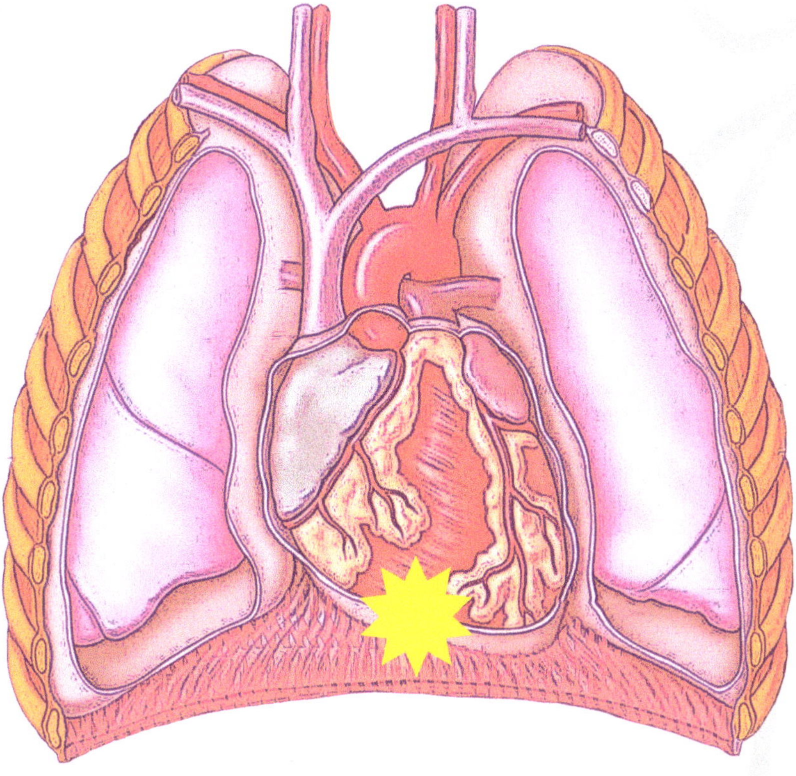

The muscle fibers of the diaphragm combine to form a central tendon. This tendon ascends to fuse with the inferior surface of the fibrous pericardium.

P
Perineum

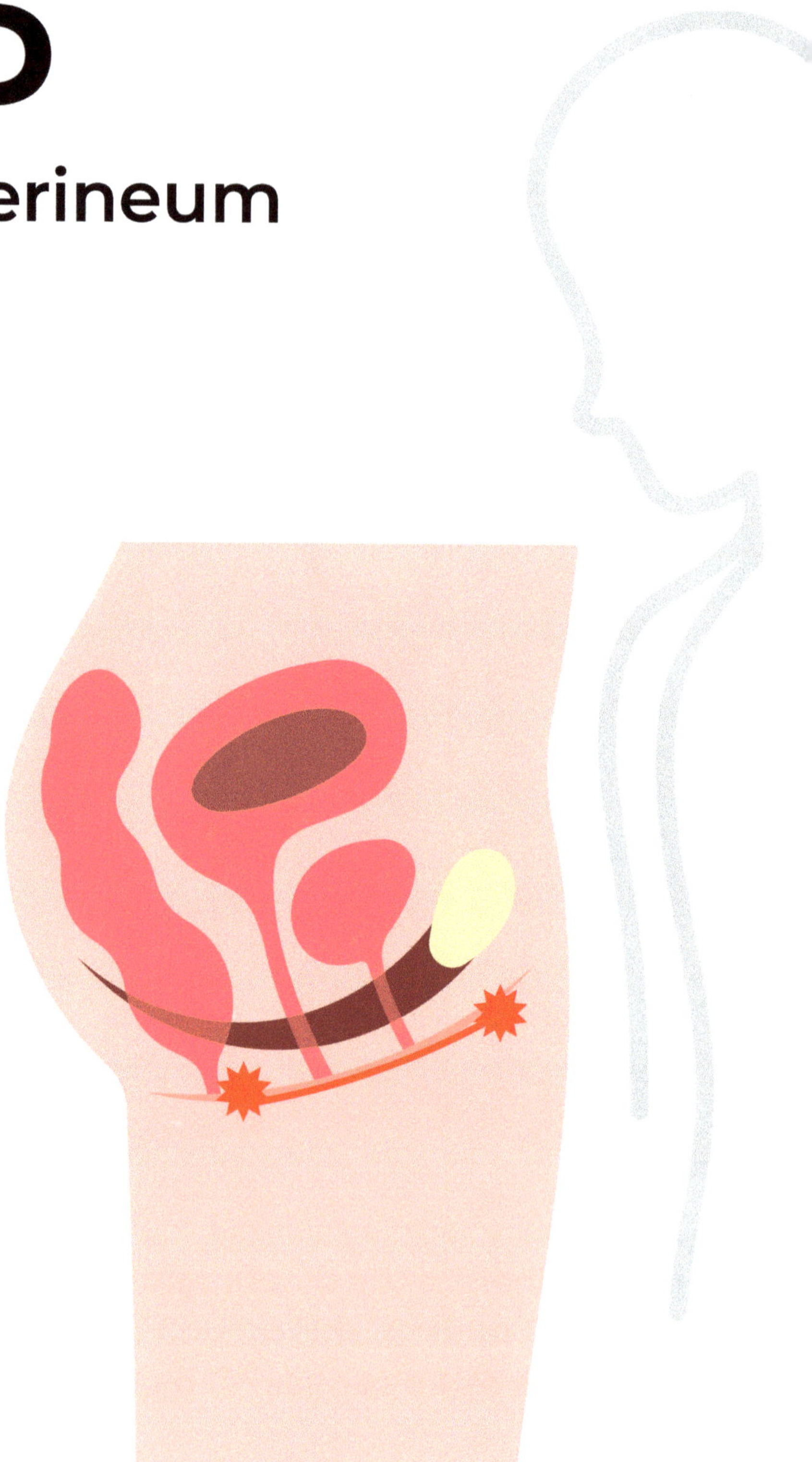

P

Piriformis (muscle)

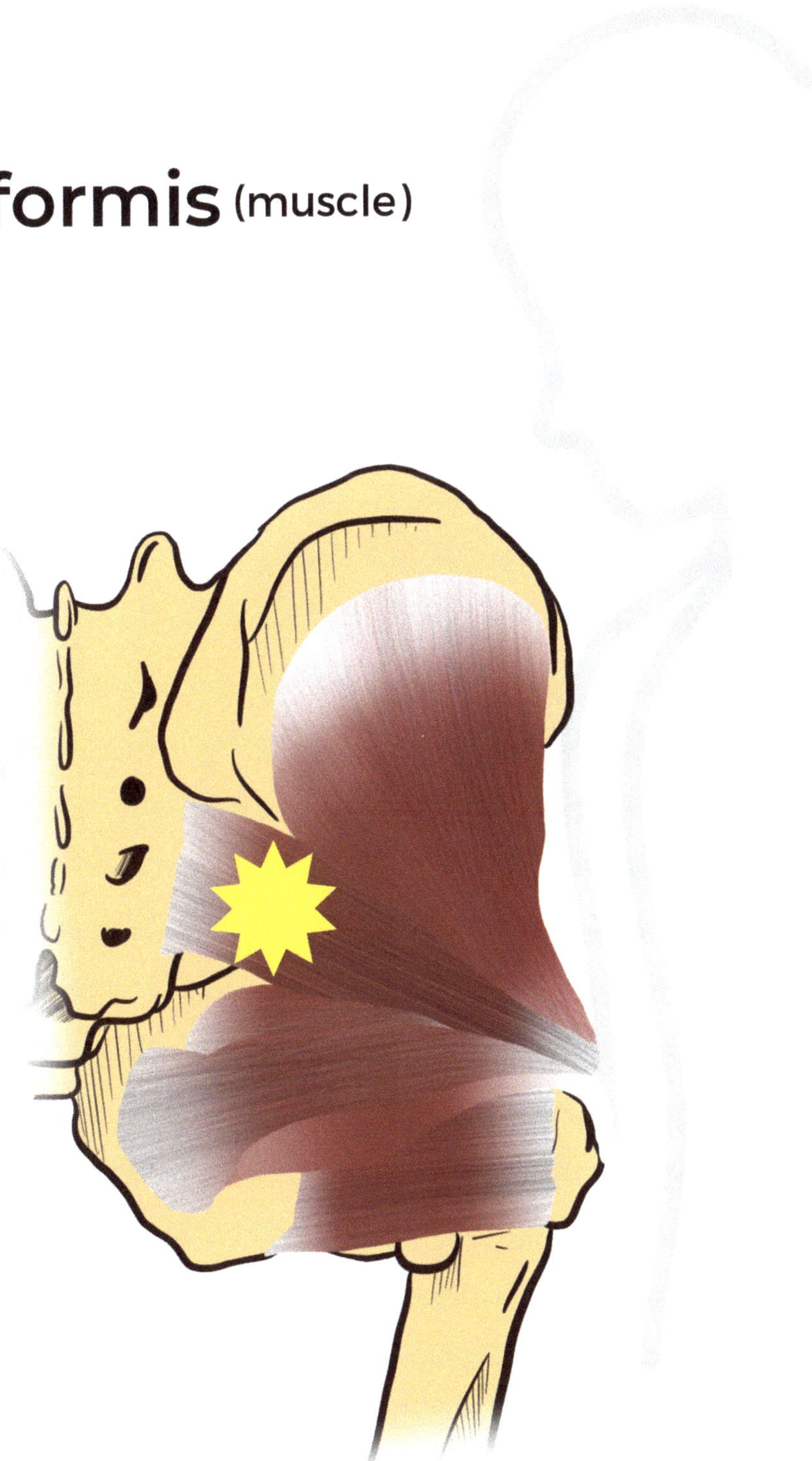

P

Pronator Teres muscle

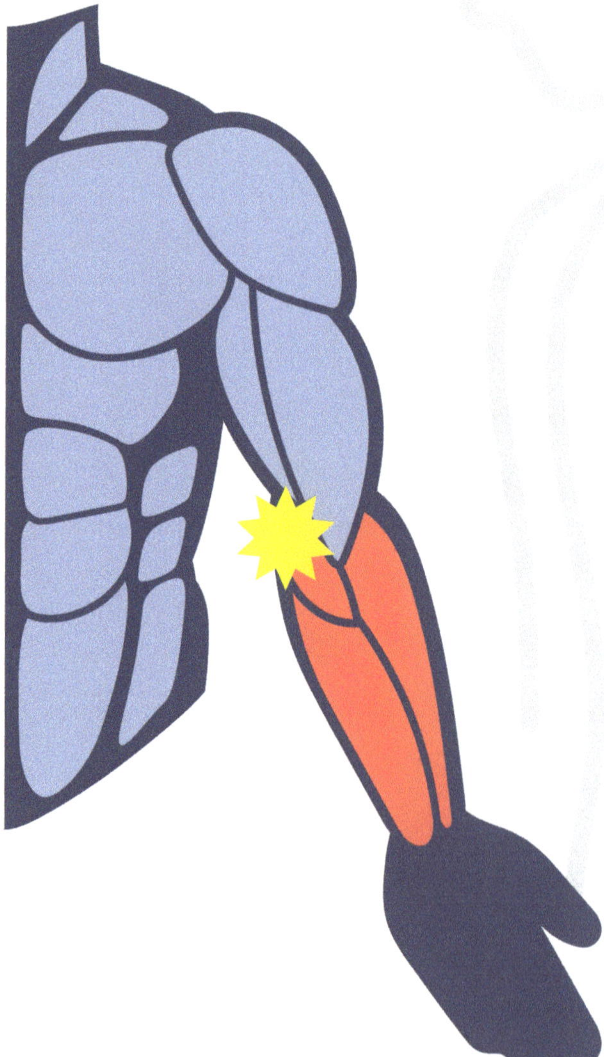

P
Prostate

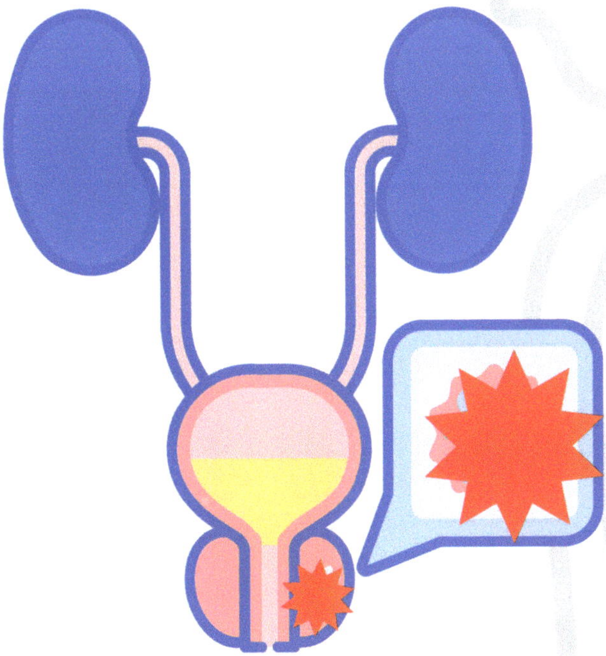

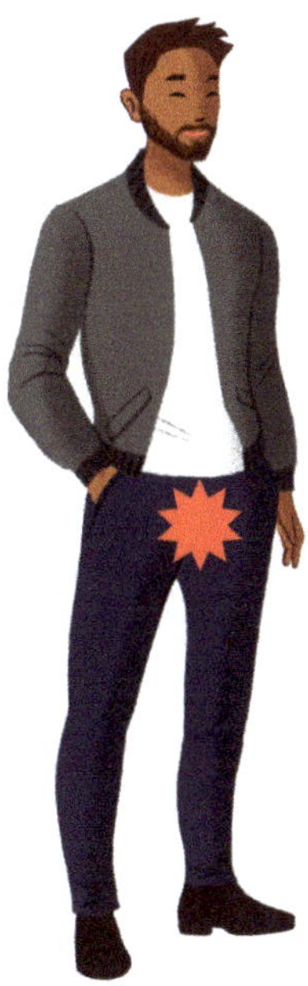

P

Psoas Major (muscle)

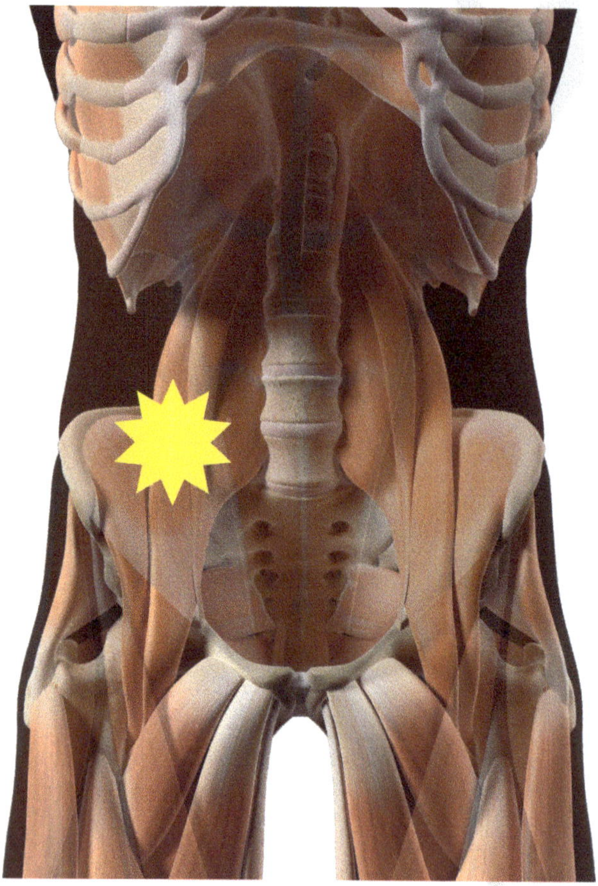

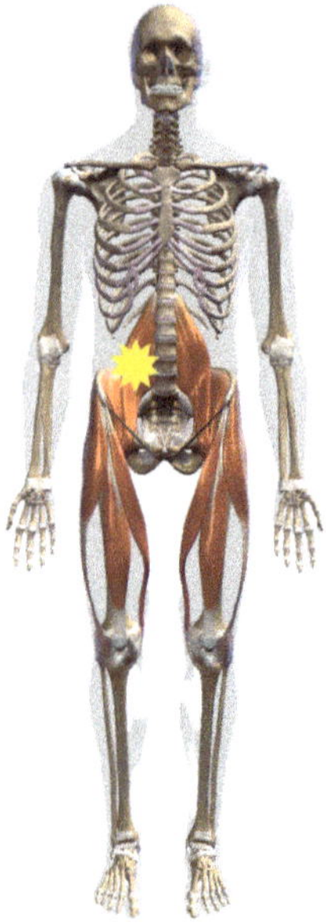

P

Pyramidalis (muscle)

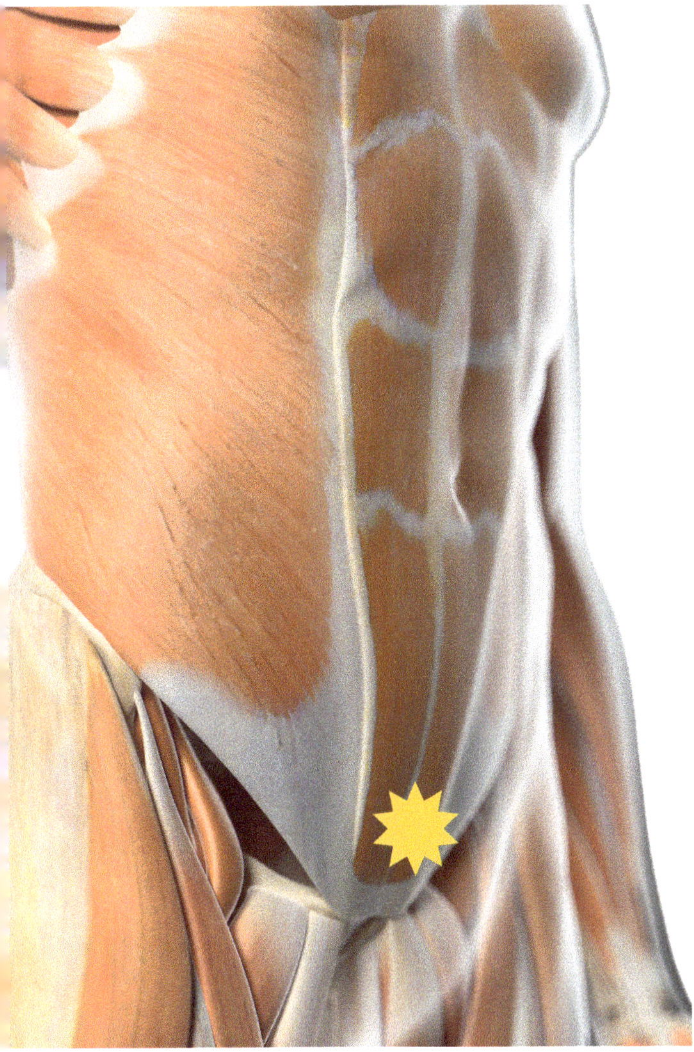

Q

Cauda Equina

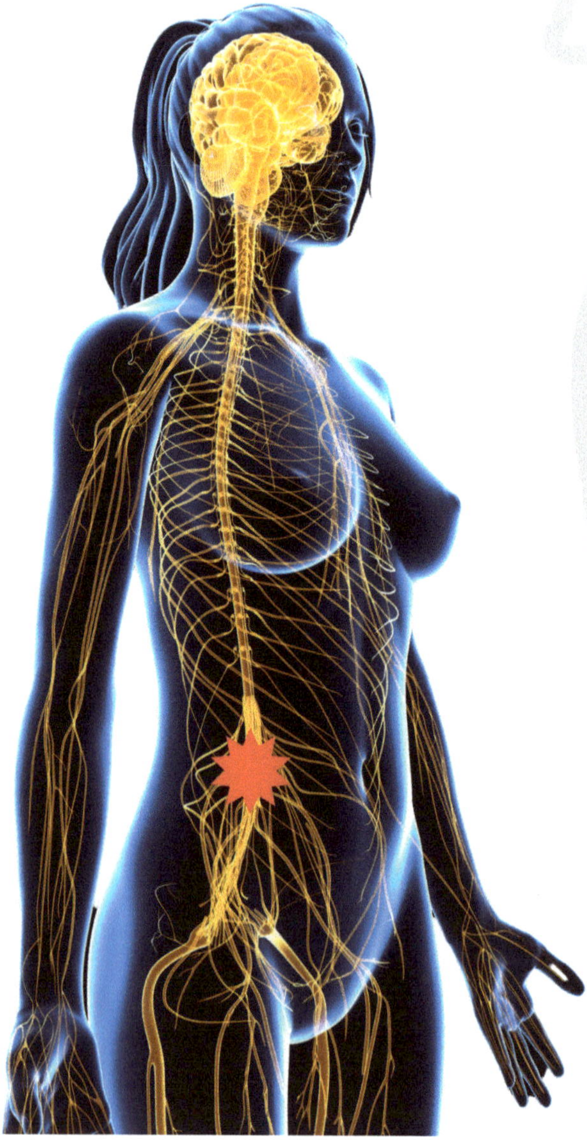

Q

Quadriceps (muscle group)

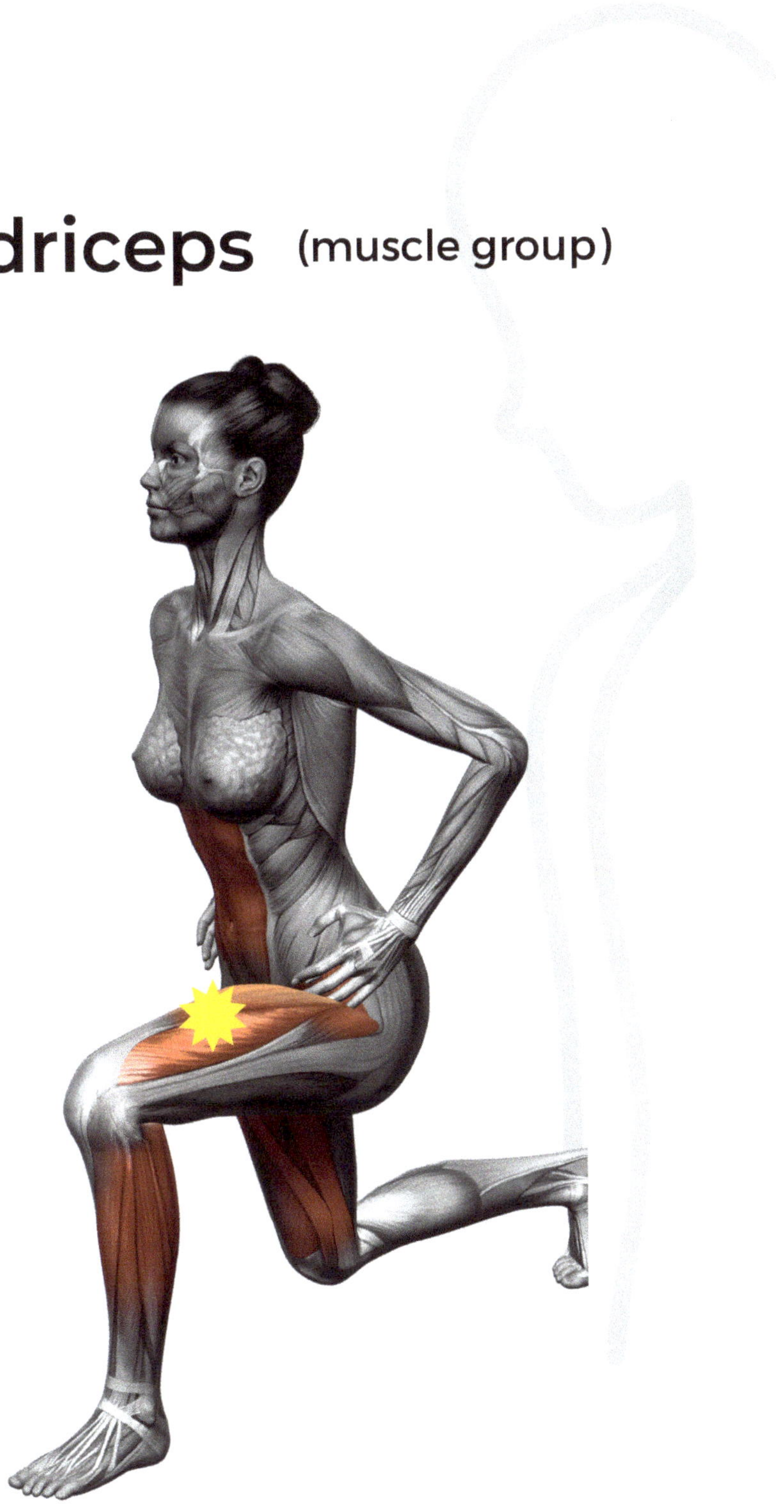

R
Rectum

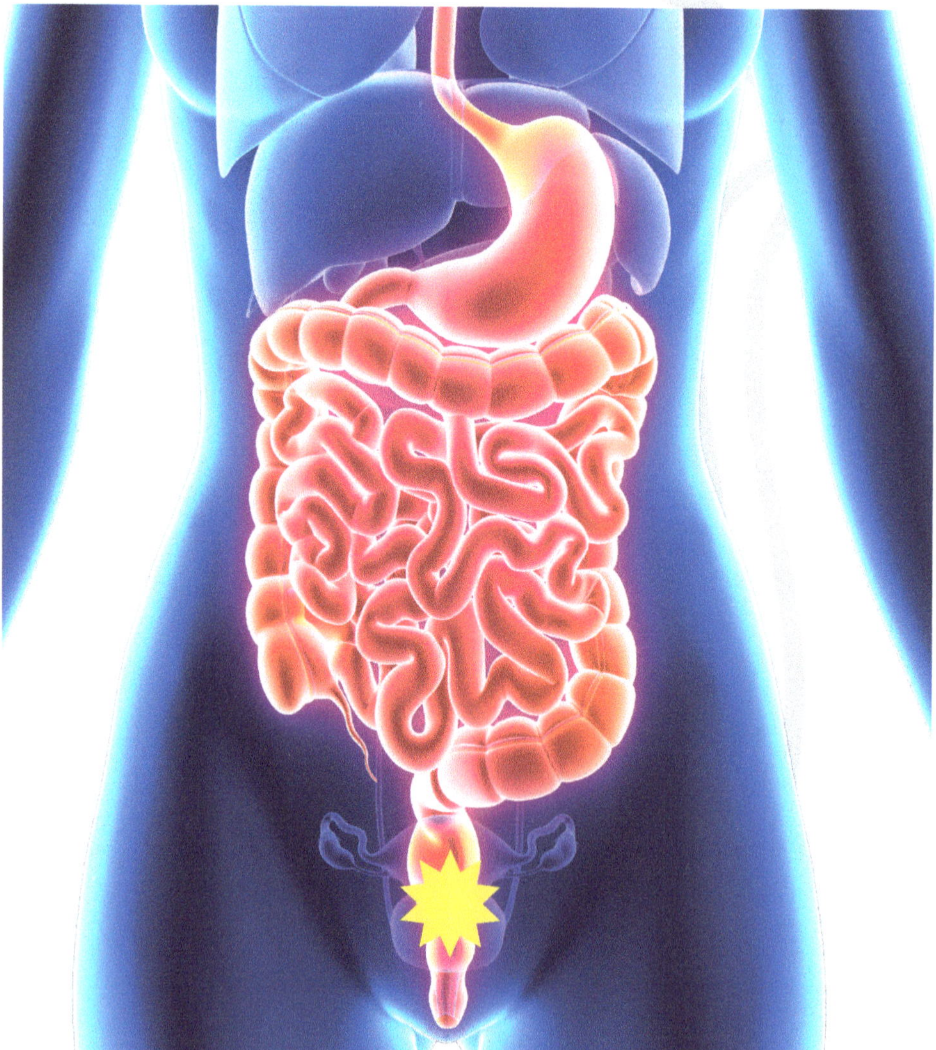

R

Rectus Abdominus (muscle)

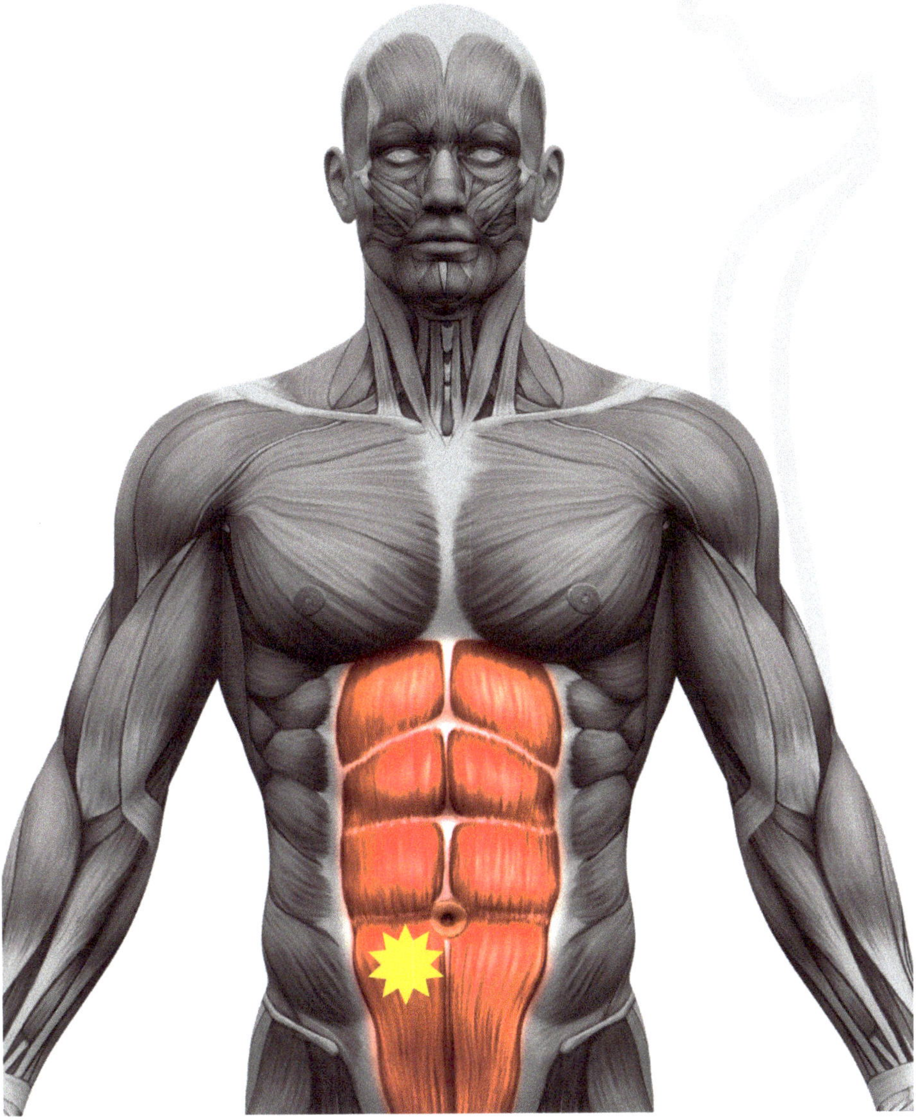

R

Rectus Femoris (muscle)

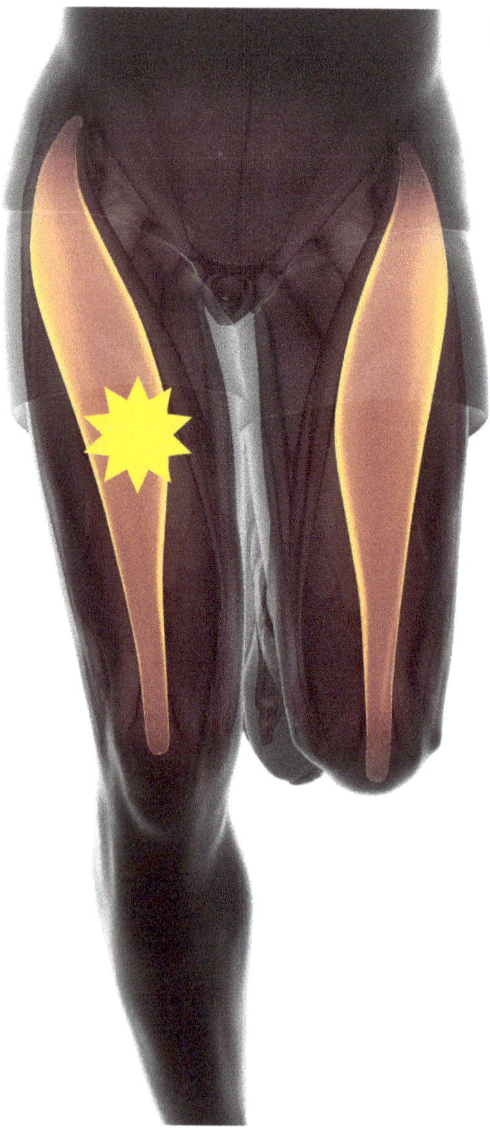

R

Round Ligament

(not pictured)

S

Scar   Skin

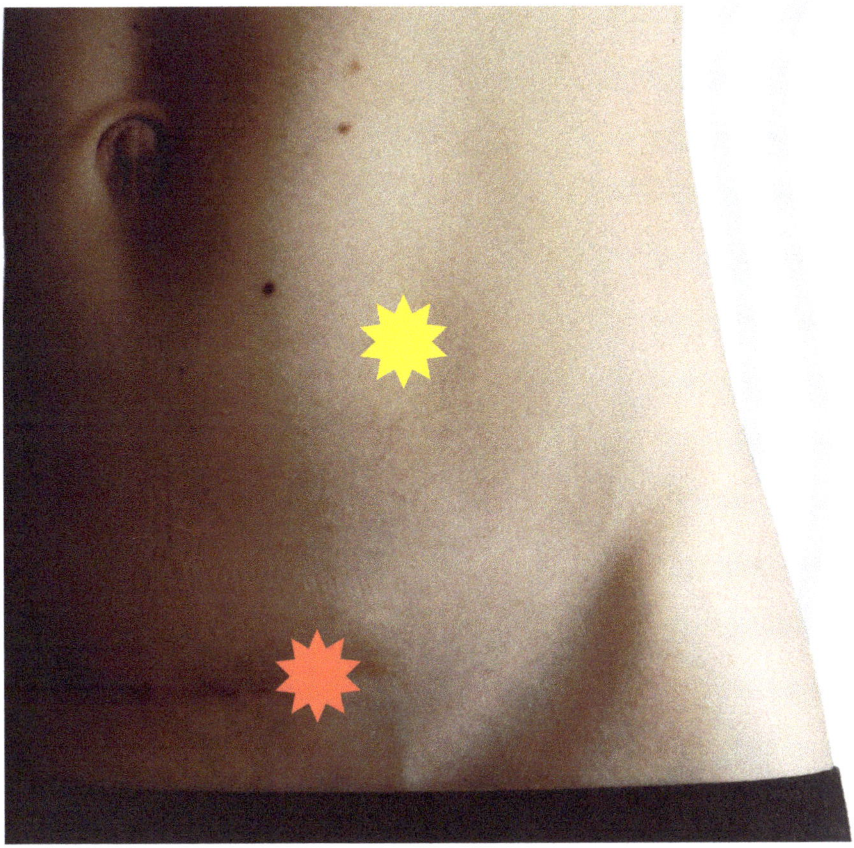

S
Sciatic Nerve

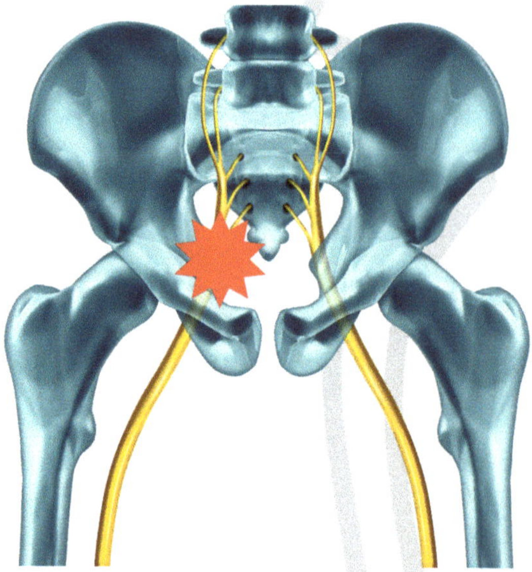

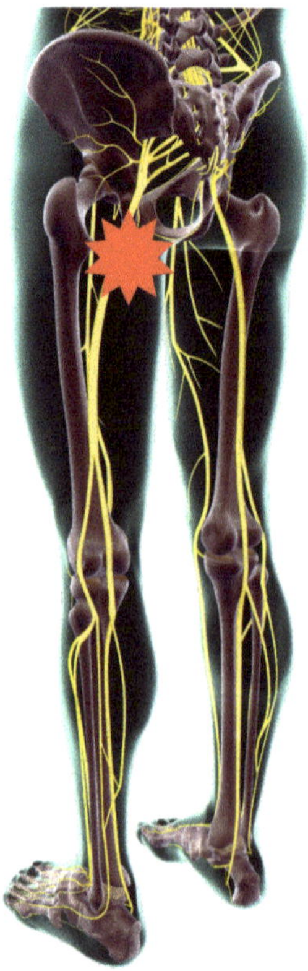

S

Semitendinosus* and Semimembranosus*

(muscle fascia)

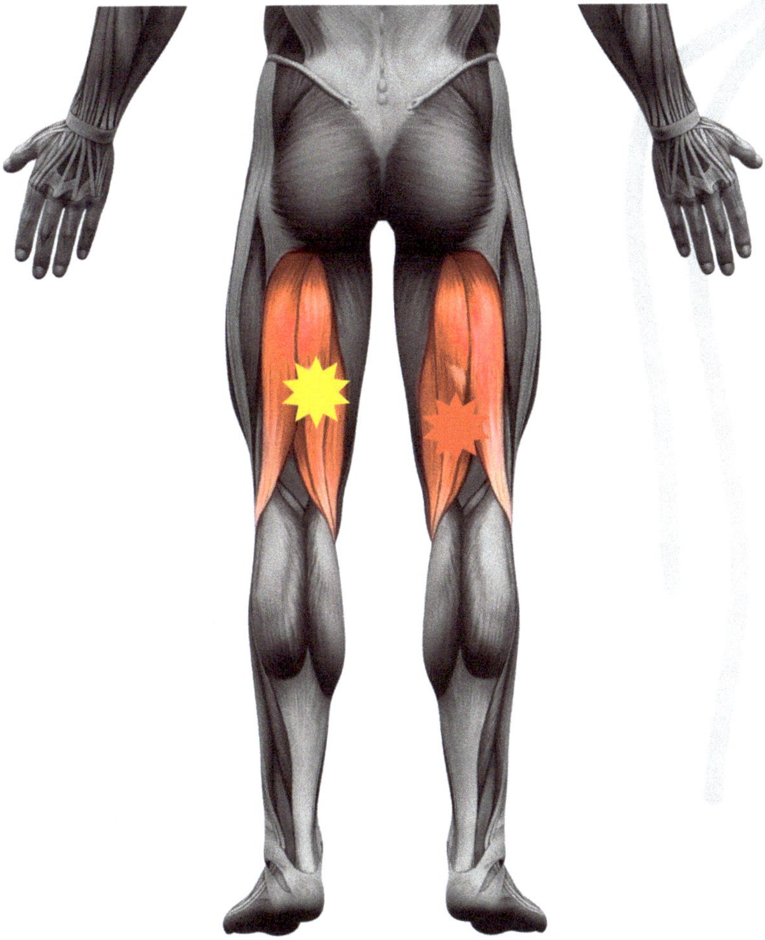

S

Sigmoid Colon

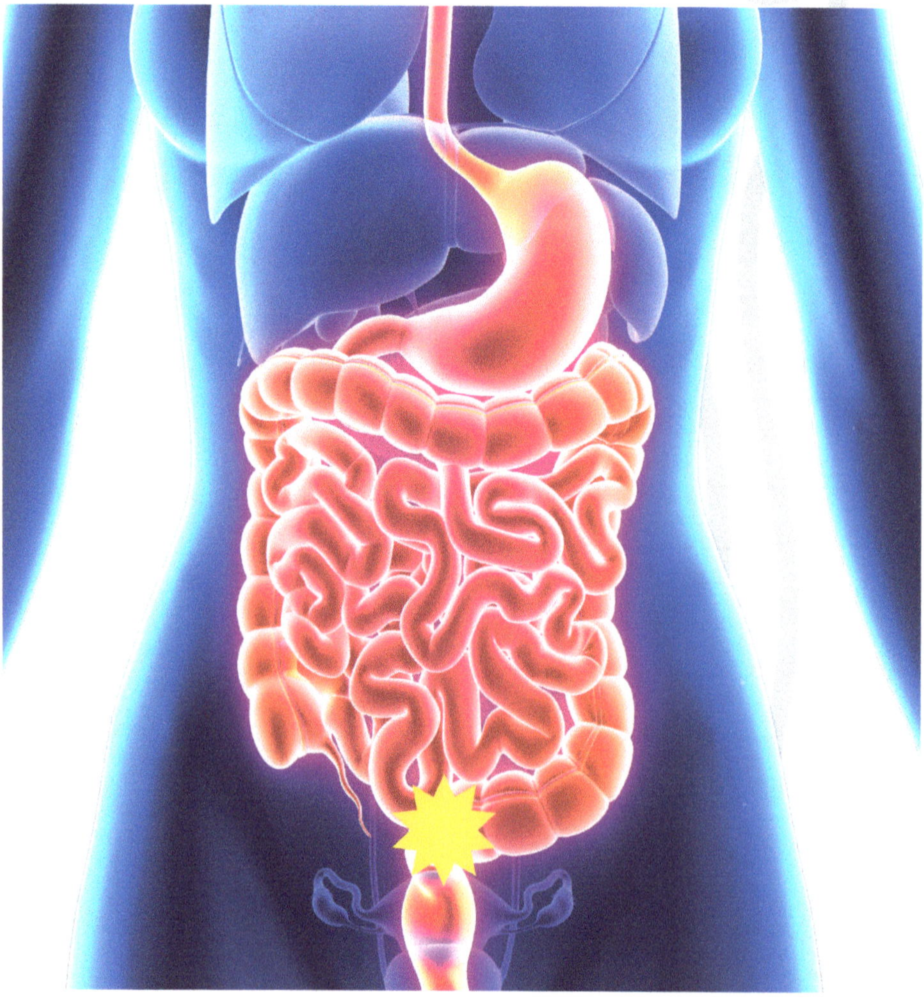

S

Soleus (muscle)

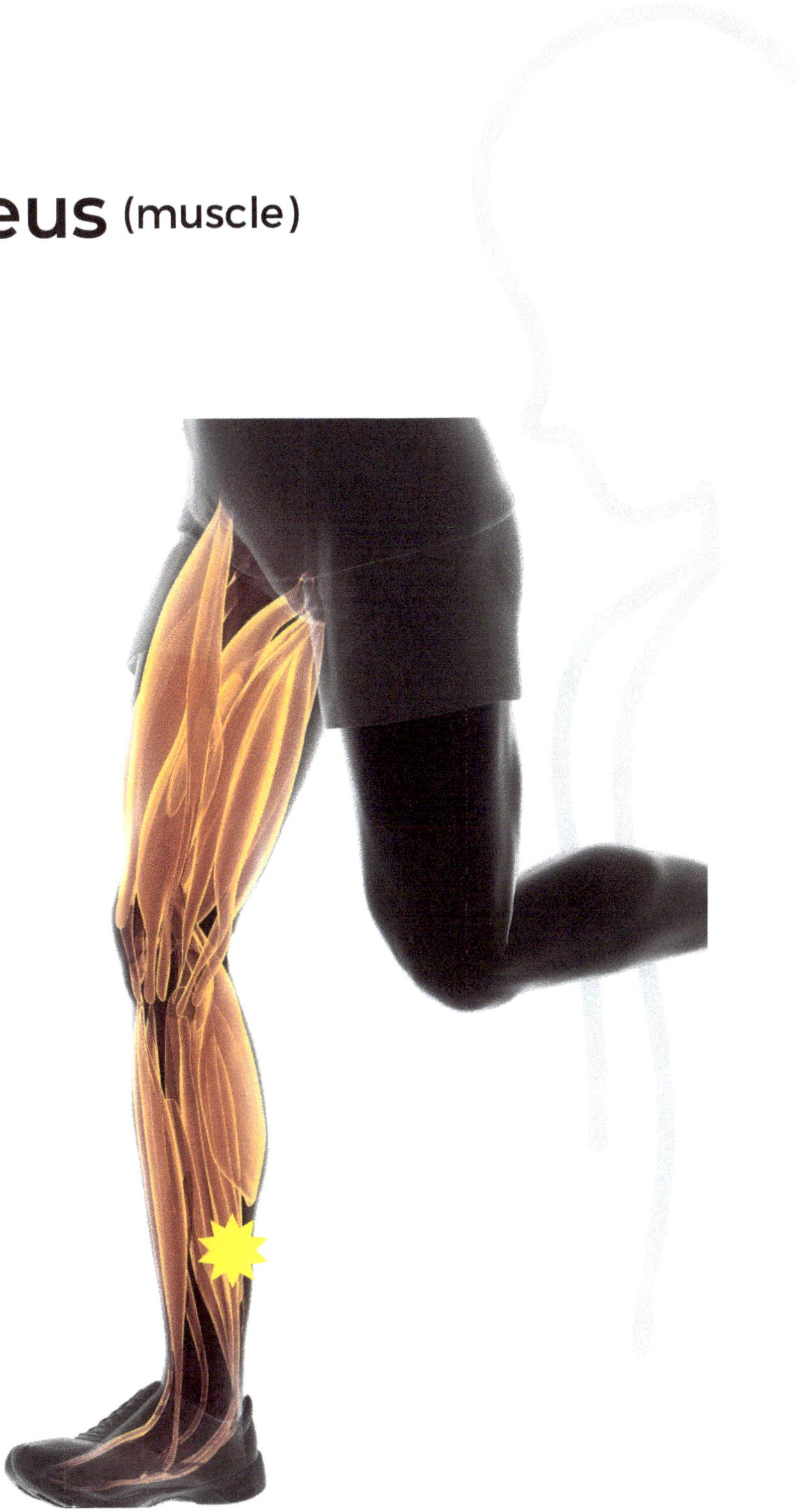

S

Spleen

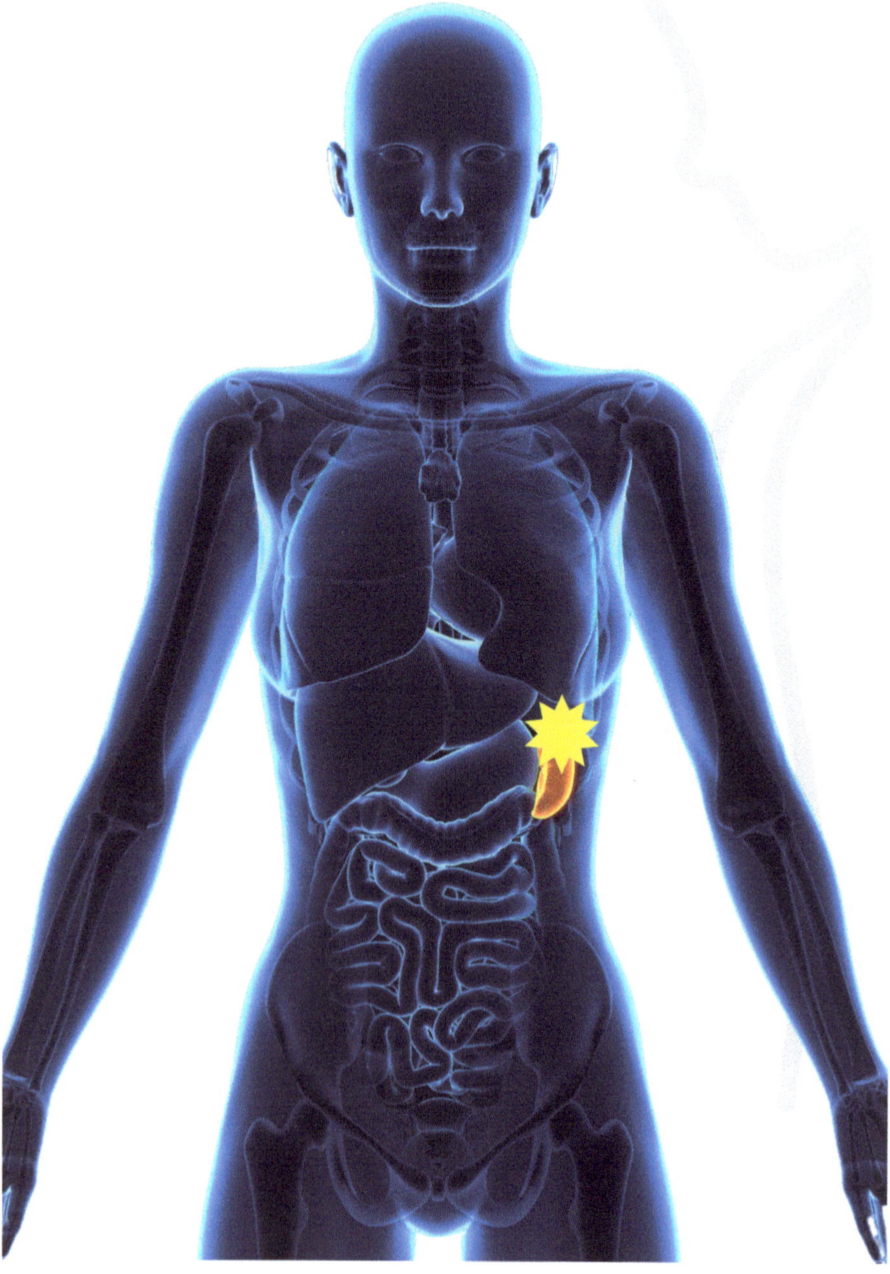

S
Stomach

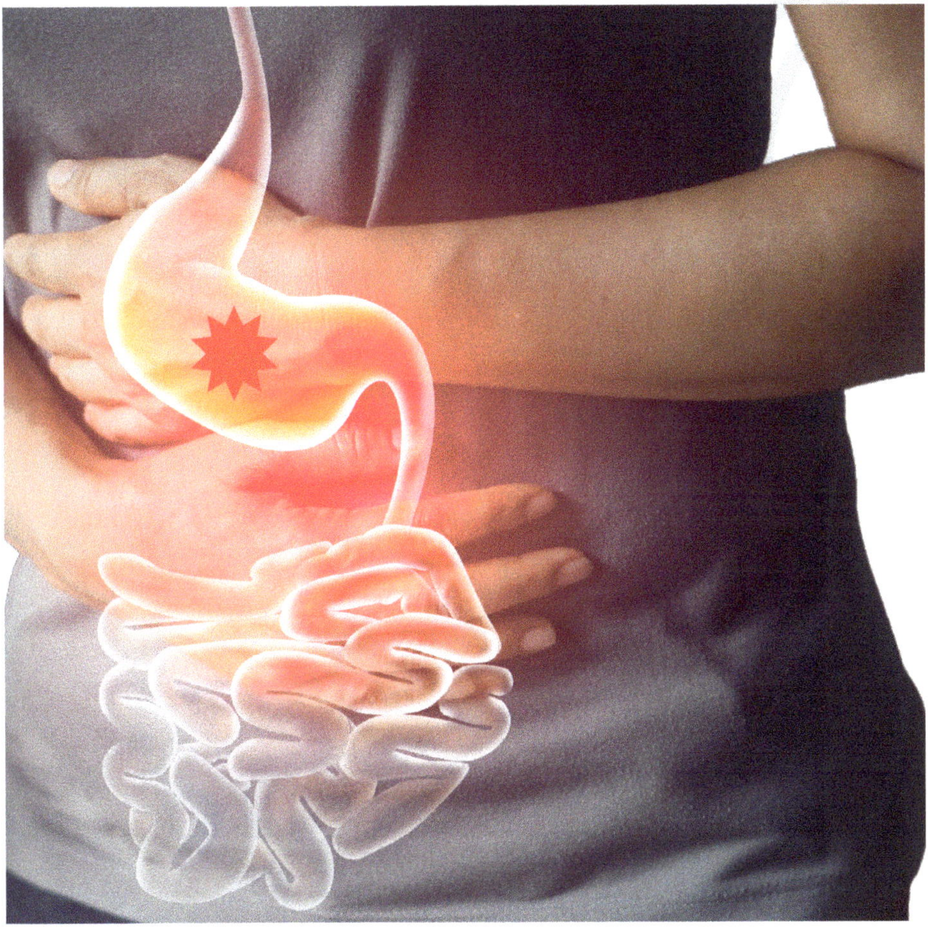

S

Subarachnoid Space

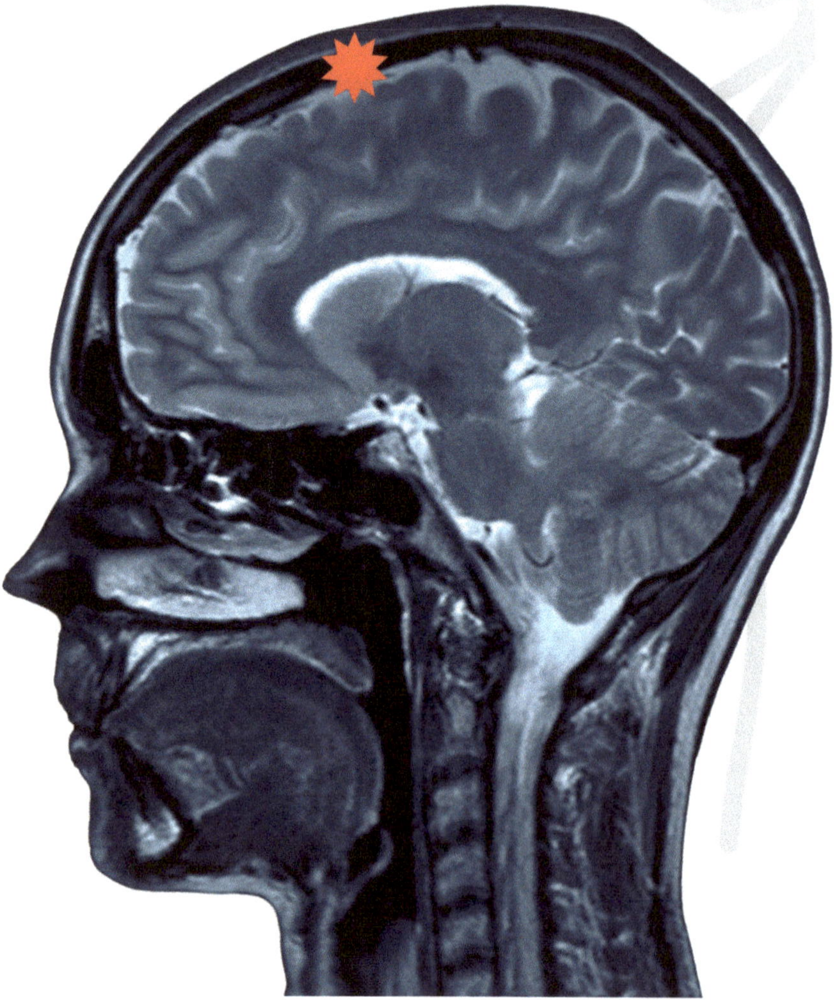

S

Superior Gluteal Nerve

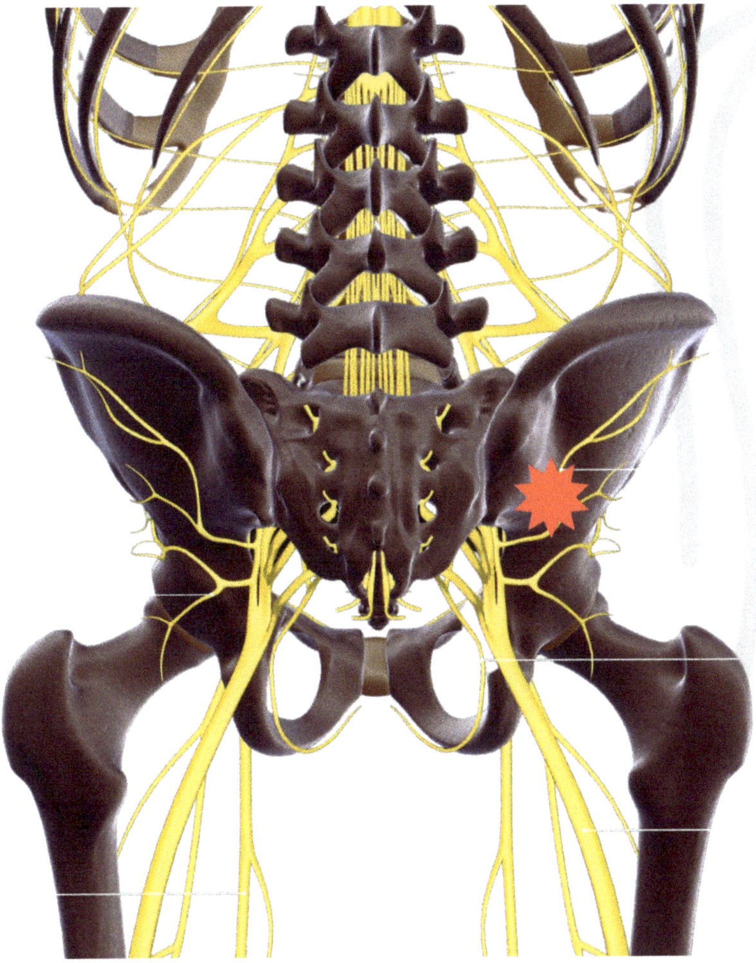

T
Testicle

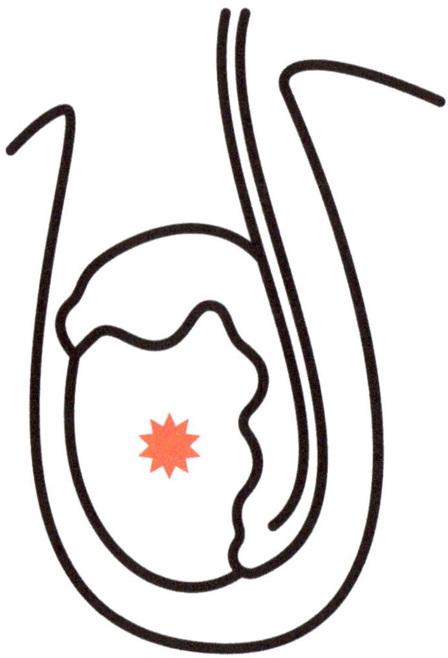

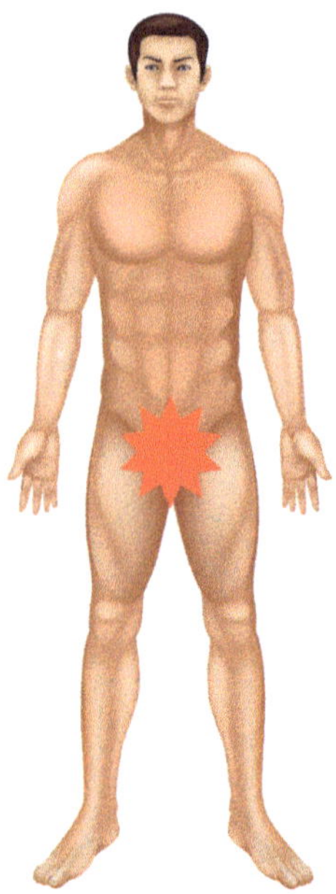

T

Thumb

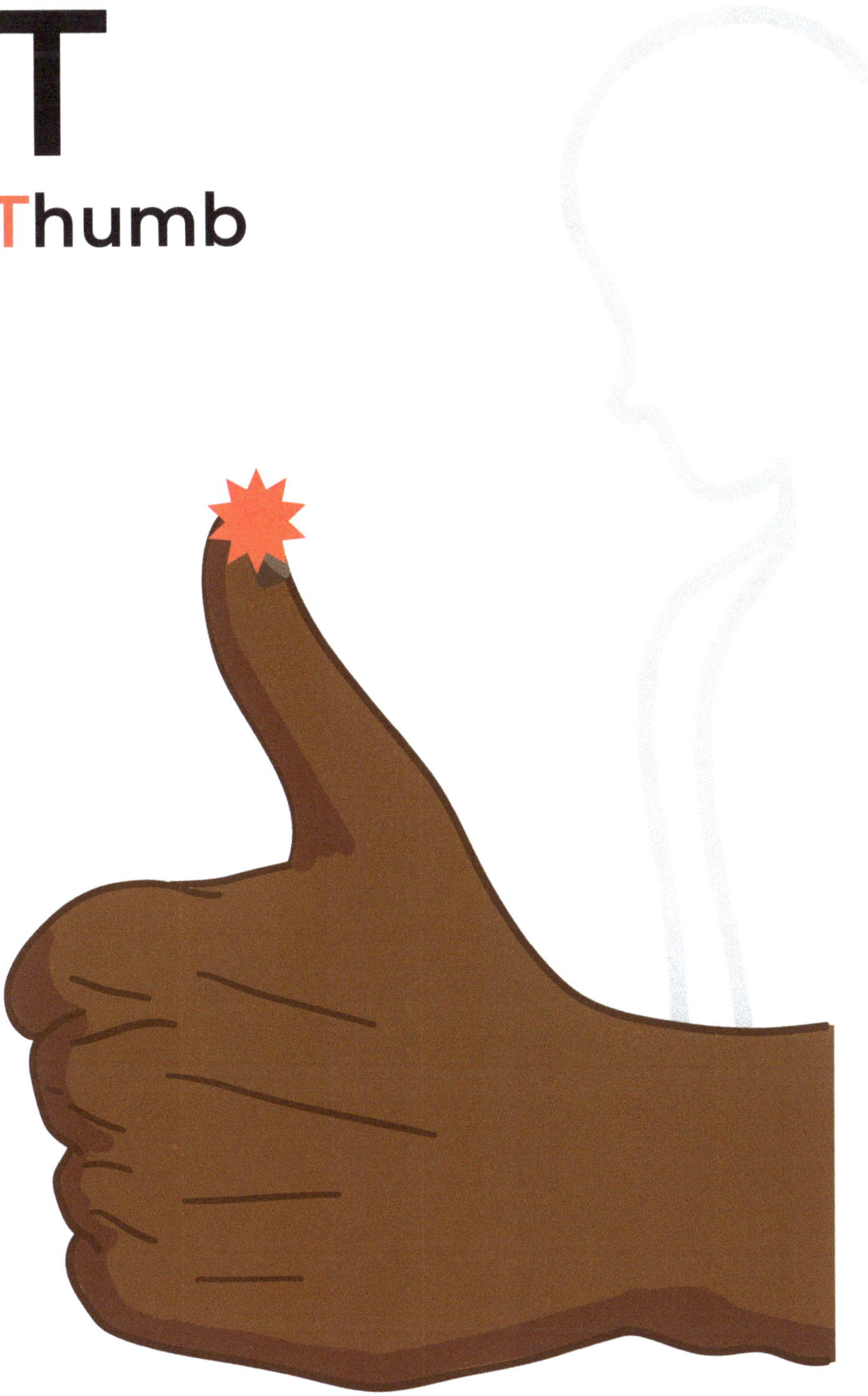

T

Trachea

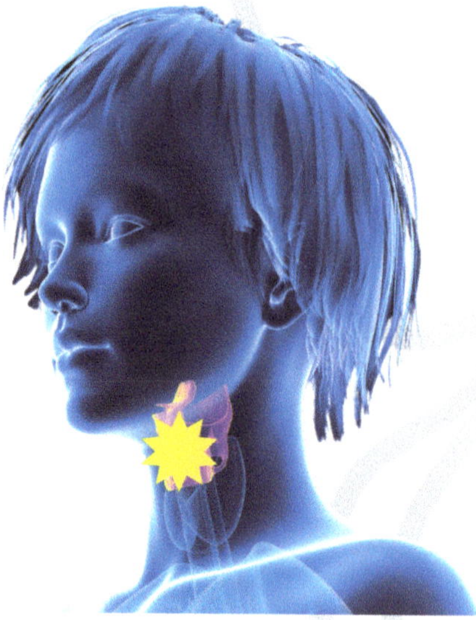

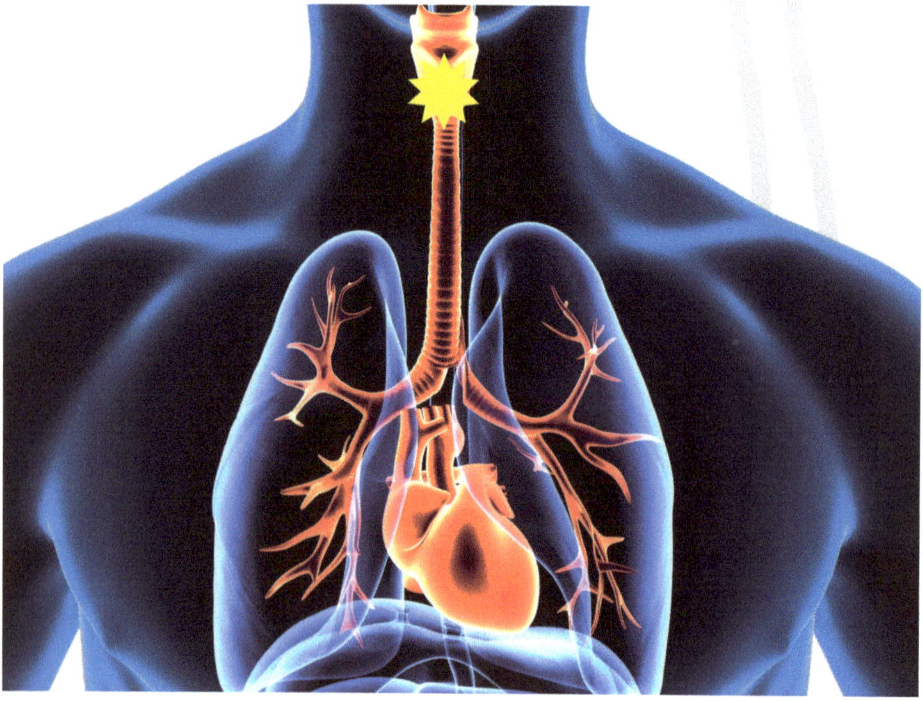

T

Transverse Colon

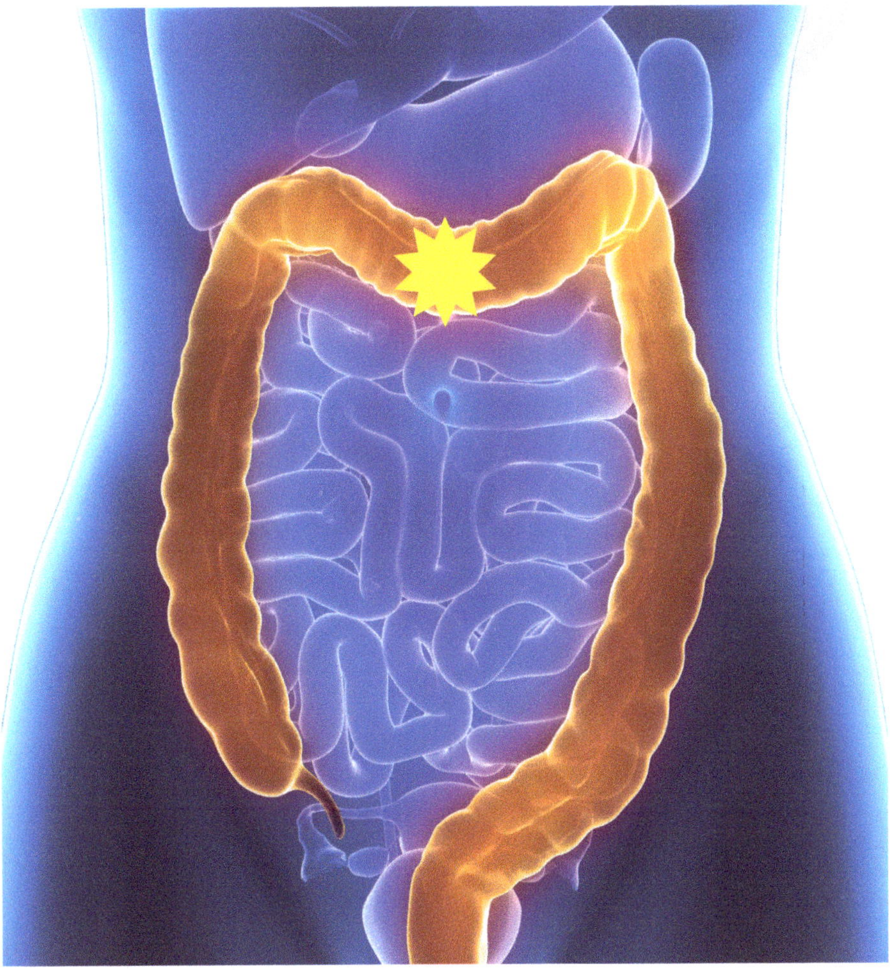

T

Trapezius (muscle)

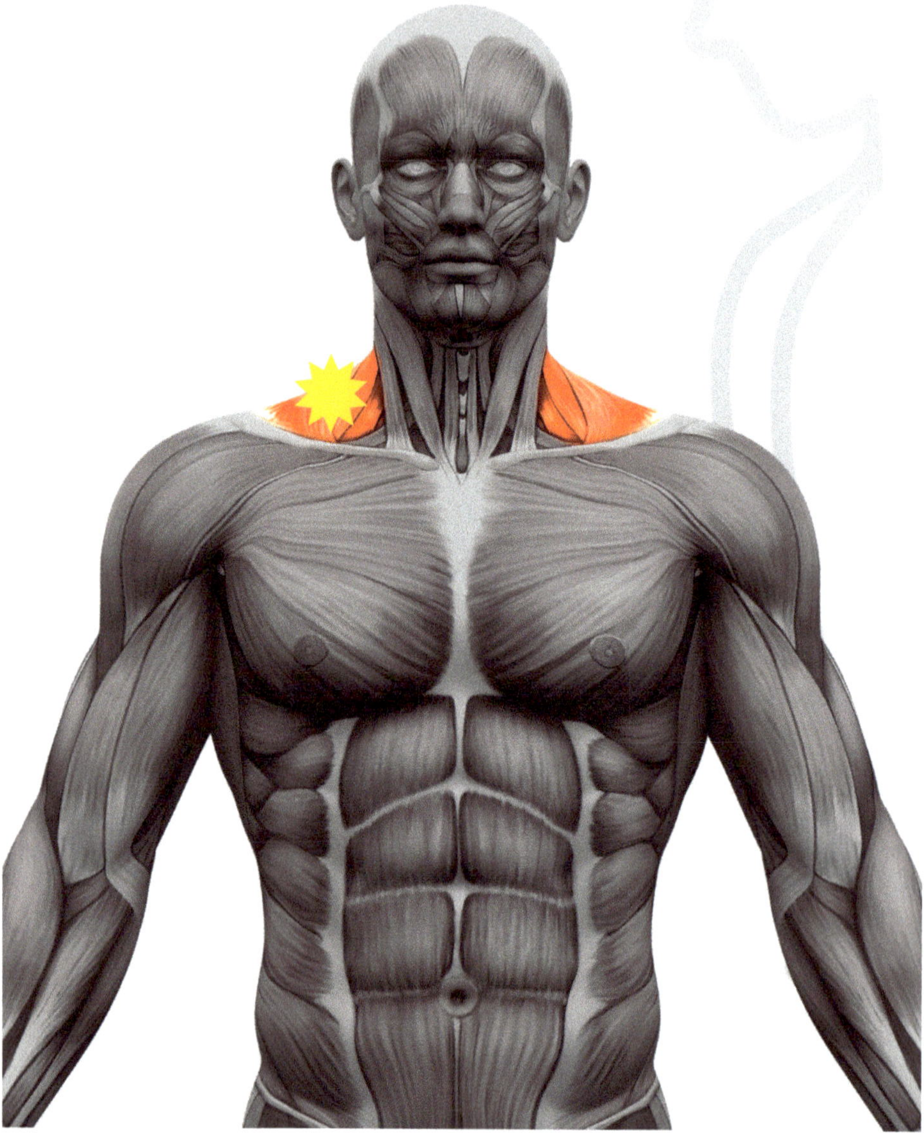

U

Umbilicus (belly button)

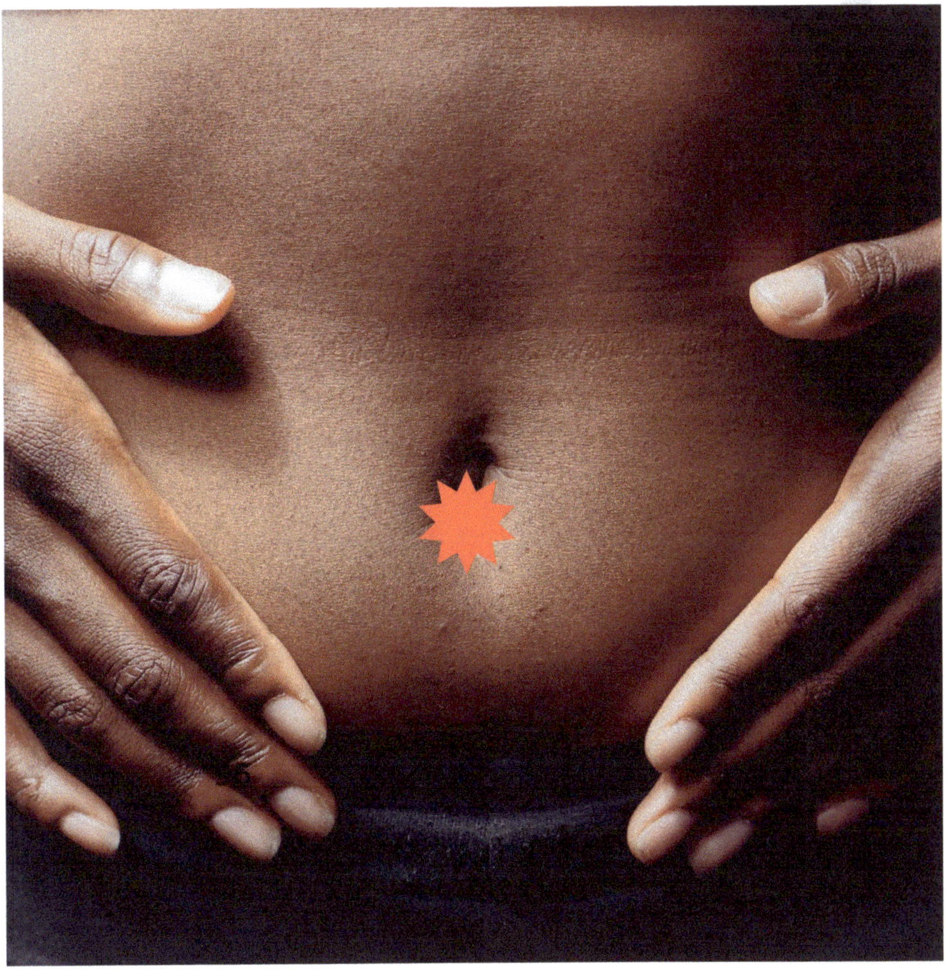

U

Ureter

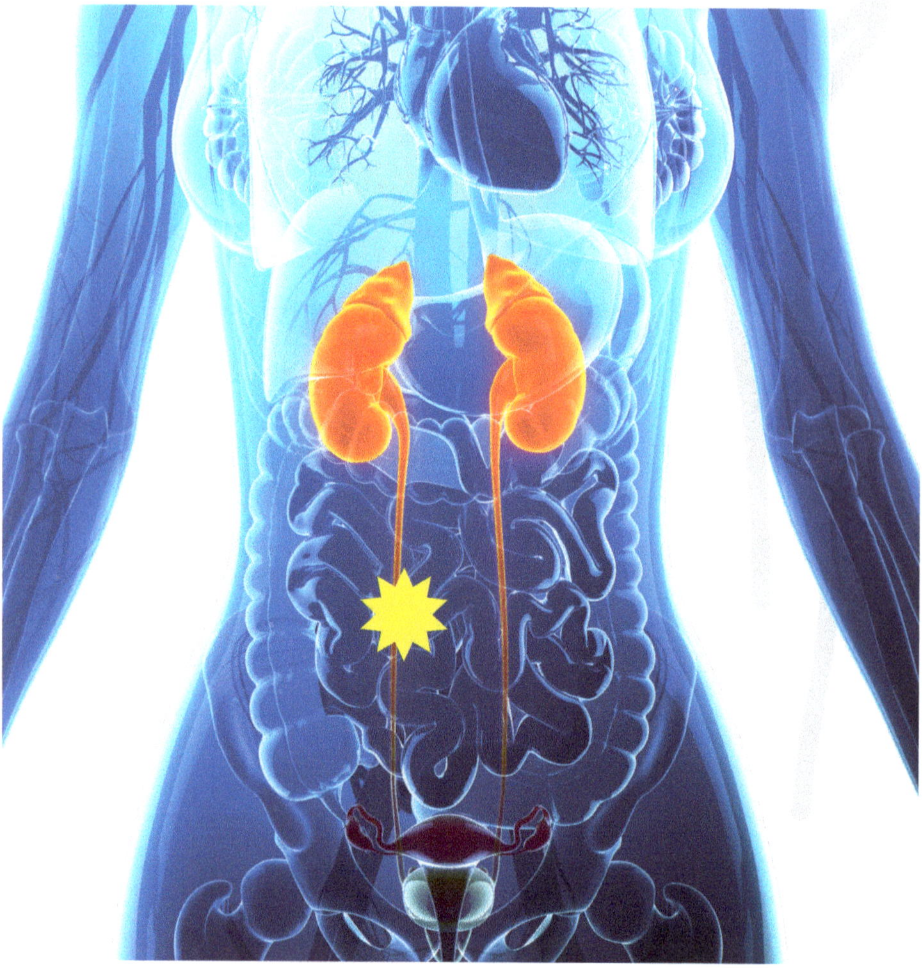

U
Urethra

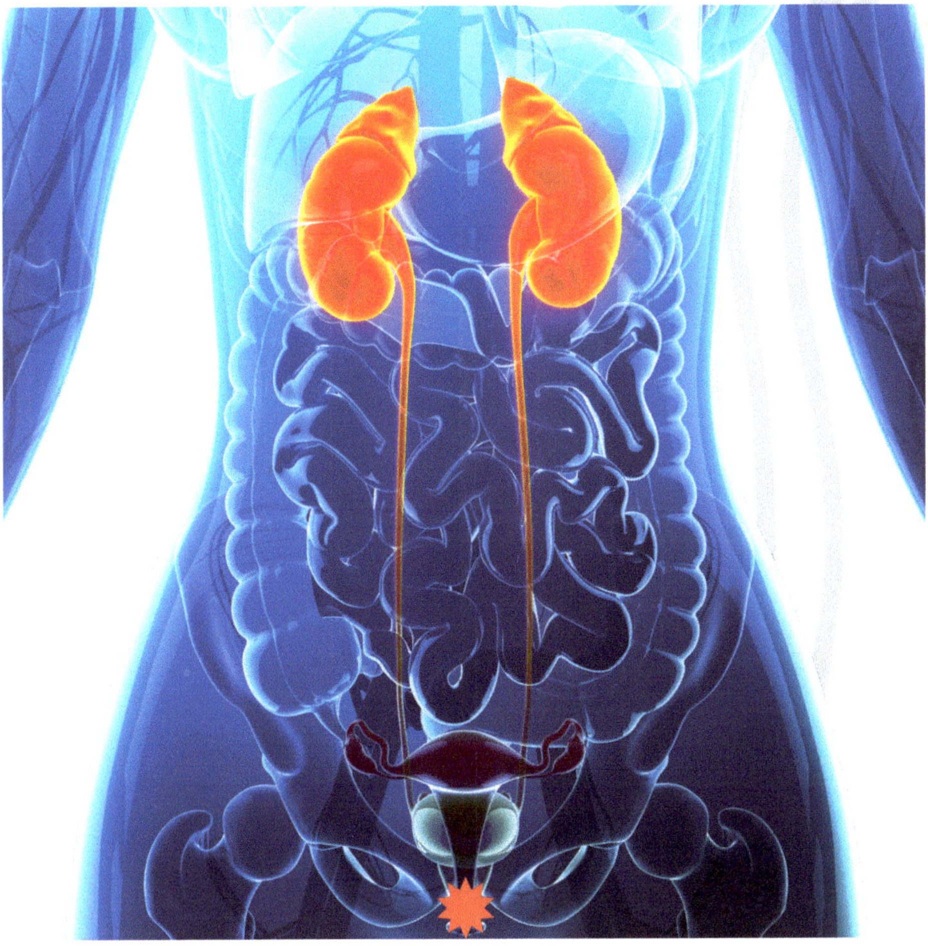

V
Vas Deferens

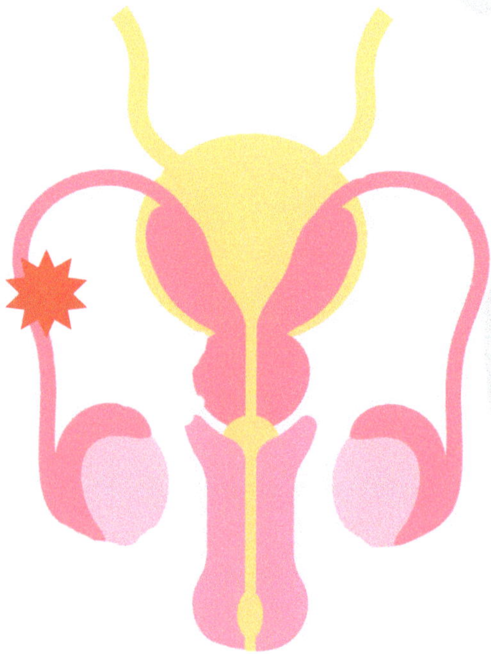

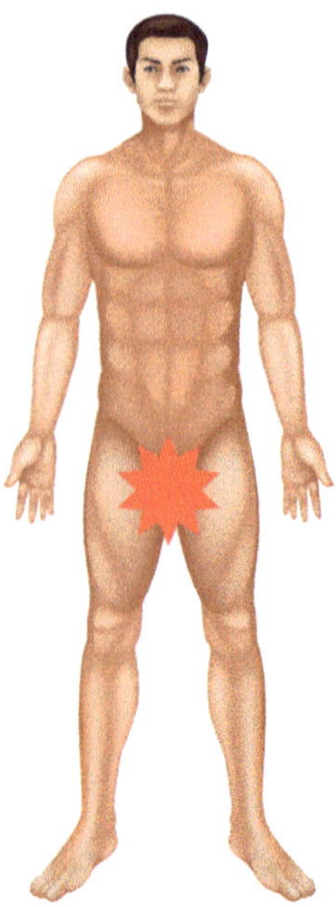

V
Vertebra

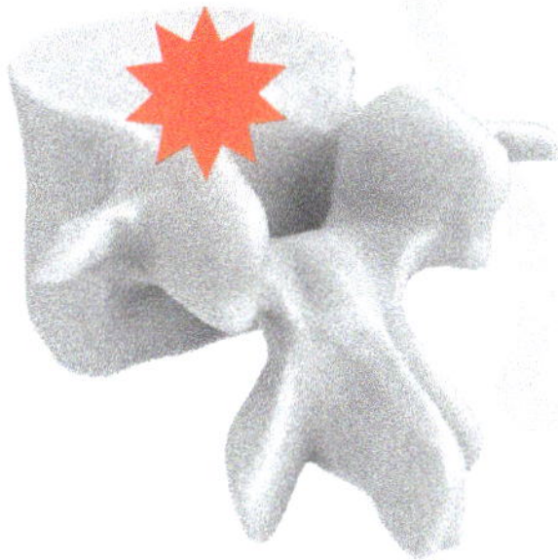

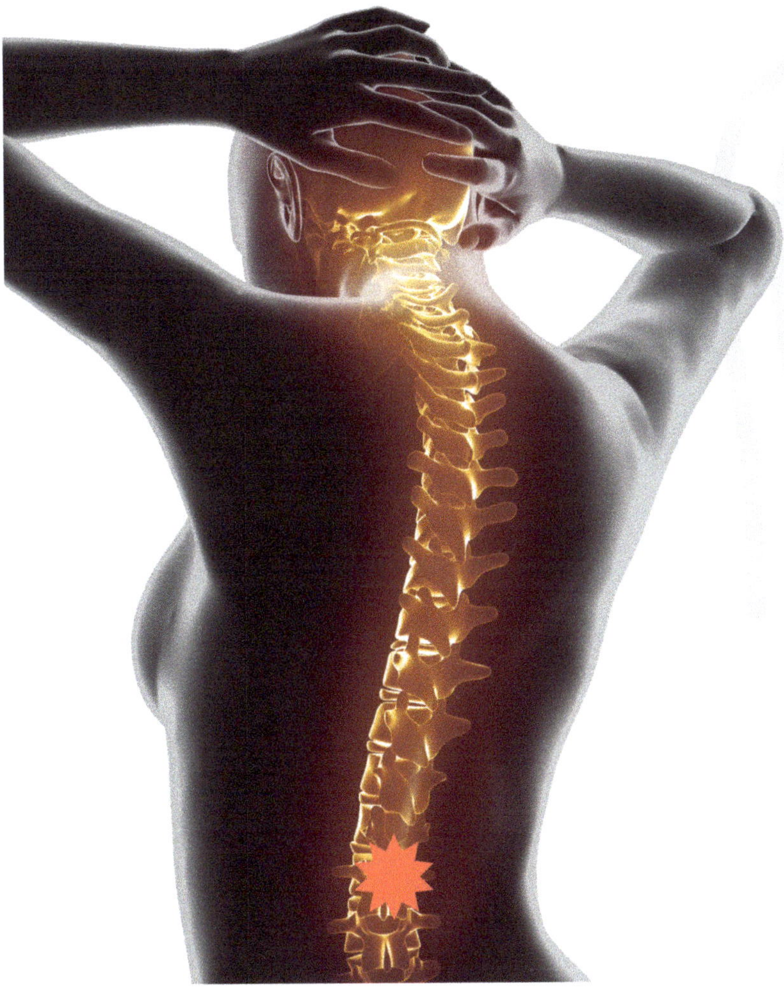

V

Visceral Pleura

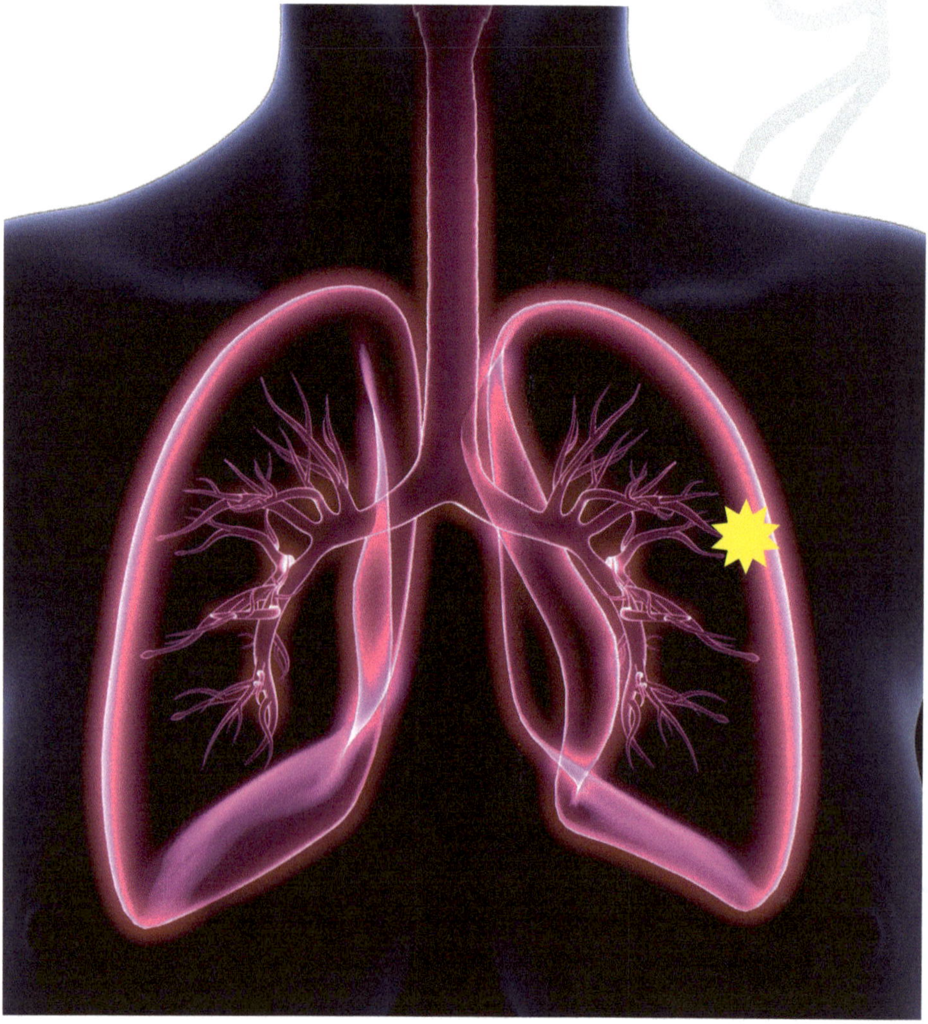

V

Vulva
Vagina

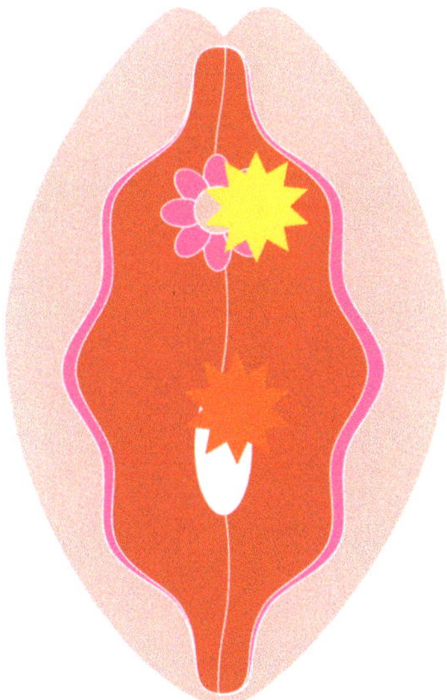

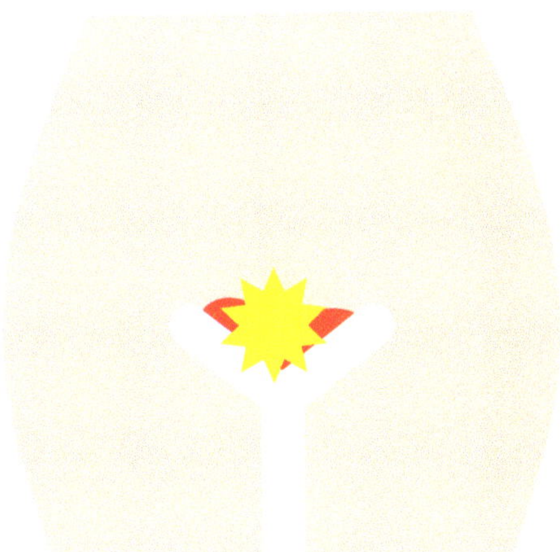

W

Wrist

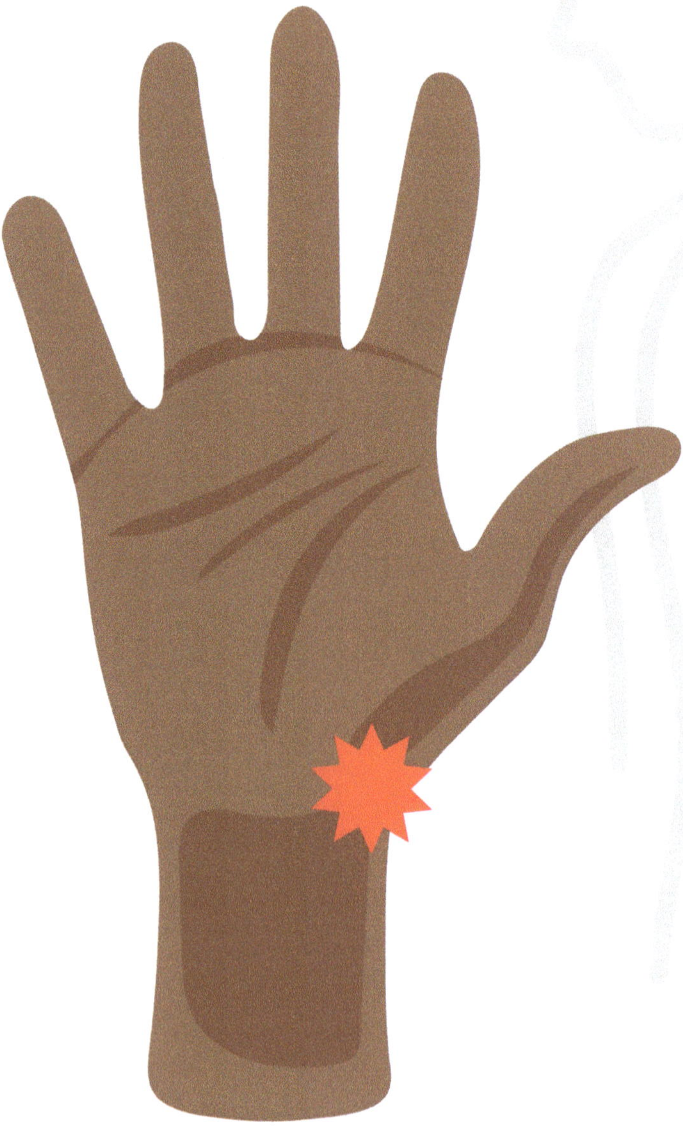

X

Sacral Plexus

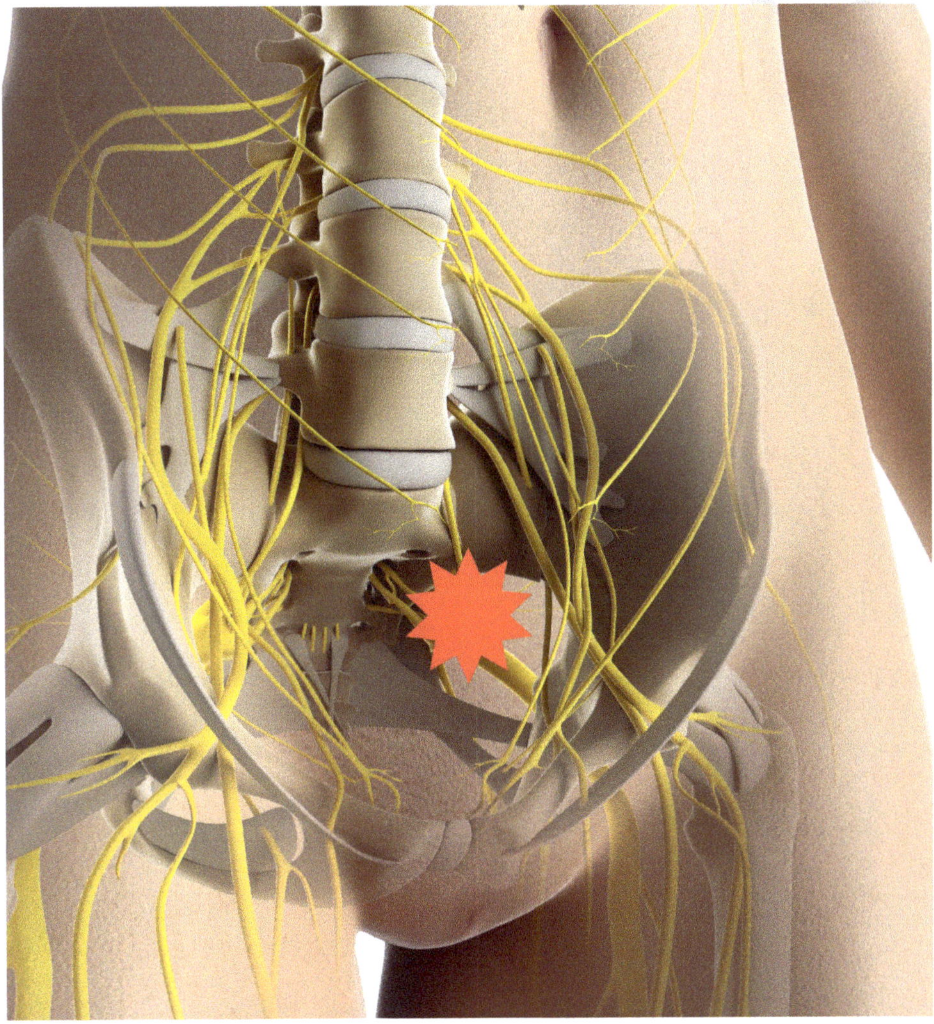

Y

Lung Parenchyma

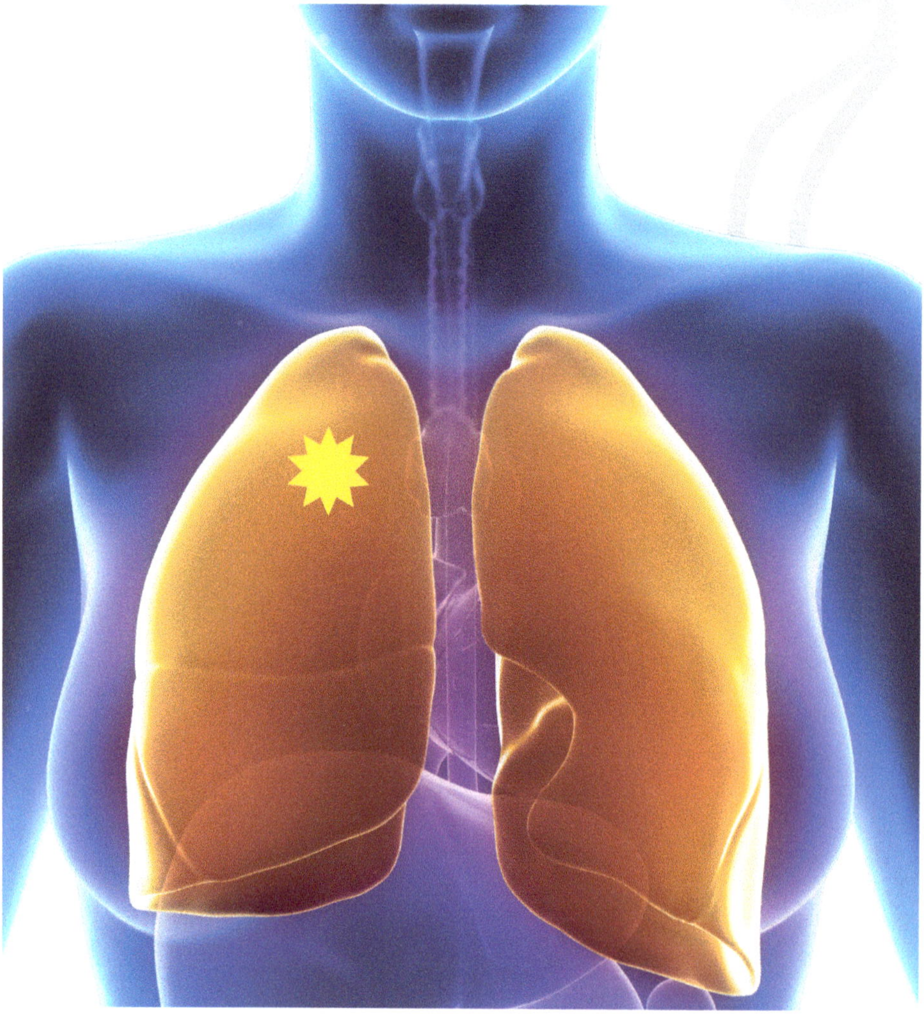

Z

Z Lines

Z Lines are components of sarcomeres.
Sarcomeres are the basic component of muscles.

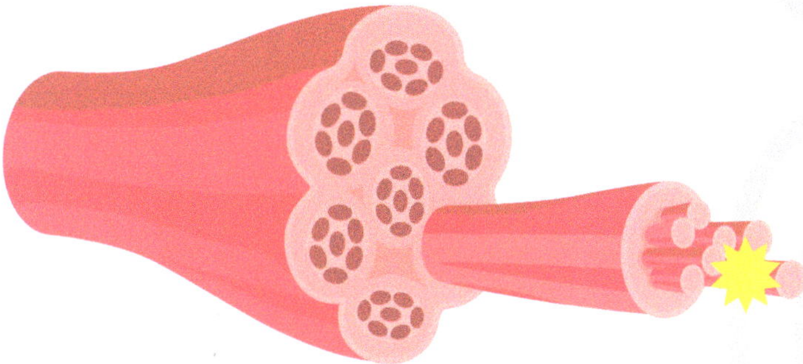

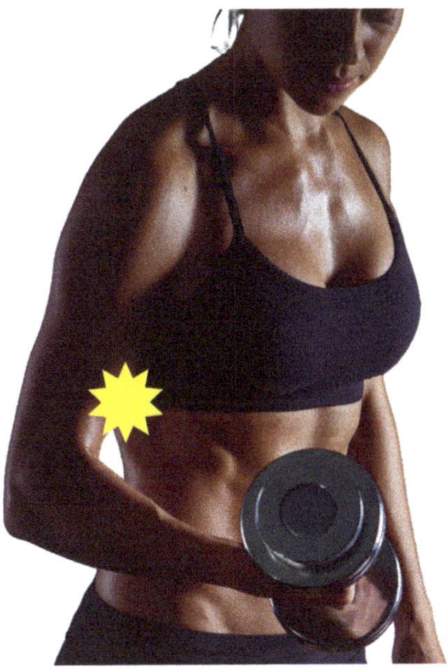

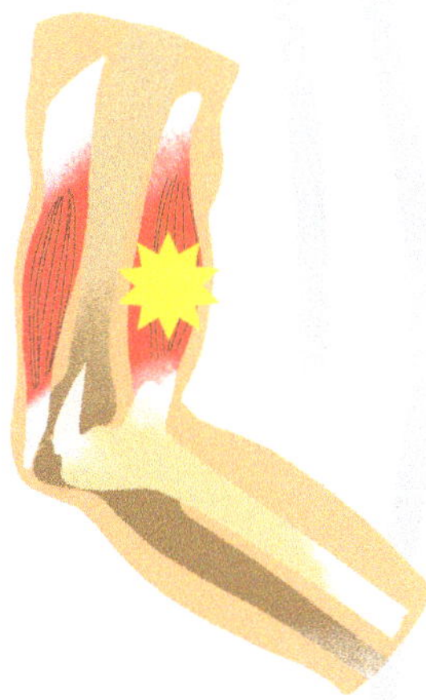

What is Extrapelvic Not Rare?

Extrapelvic Not Rare (EPNR) is a non-profit organization (NPO) based in Vancouver, Washington, USA.

EPNR's mission is to educate, advocate, conduct and support research for endometriosis as a disease with body-wide lesion potential and capacity to disrupt systemic homeostasis.

EPNR does not receive funding from pharmaceutical or associated companies that financially benefit from products or services associated with the disease.

More information about EPNR and endometriosis of nonreproductive tissues or make a financial contribution to support our mission:

extrapelvicnotrare.org

Citations

Did You Know?

A to Z

Citations
Did You Know?

1. Klemmt PAB, Starzinski-Powitz A. Molecular and Cellular Pathogenesis of Endometriosis. Current Women's Health Review.2018;14: 106-116.Doi:10.2174/1573404813666170306163448

2. Lagana AS, Garzon S, Gotte M, Vigano P, Franchi M, Gheezzi F, Marti DC. The Pathogenesis of Endometriosis: Molecular and Cell Biology Insights. Int J Mol Sci.2019;20(22): 5615. Doi: 10.3390/ijms20225615

3. Vercellini, P., Viganò, P., Somigliana, E. et al. Endometriosis: pathogenesis and treatment. Nat Rev Endocrinol 10, 261–275 (2014). https://doi.org/10.1038/nrendo.2013.255

4. Boyle DP, McCluggae WG. Peritoneal Stromal Endometriosis: a detailed morphological analysis of a large series of cases of a common and under-recognized form of endometriosis. J Clin Pathol. 2009;62:530-533. Doi: 10.1136/jcp.2008.06426

Citations
Did You Know?

5. Stegmann BJ, Sinaii N, Liu S, Segars J, Merino M, Nieman LK, Stratton P. Using Location, Color Size, and Depth to Characterize and Idenfity Endometriosis Lesions in a Cohort of 133 Women. Fertil Steril.2008;89(6):1632-1636.

6. Stratton P, Winkel CA, Sinaii N, Merino MJ, Zimmer C, Nieman LK. Location, color, size, depth, and volume may predict endometriosis in lesions resected at surgery. Fertil Steril.2002;78:743–9.

7. Stripling MC, Martin DC, Chatman DL, Zwaag RV, Poston WM. Subtle appearance of pelvic endometriosis. Fertil Steril. 1988;49: pp.427–31. Doi:10.1016/s0015-0282(16)59767-2

8. Martin D, Redwine D, Reich H, Kresch AJ. Laparoscopic Appearance of Endometriosis. Second Edition, Vol.1. 1990. Resurge Press. Richmond, VA. Copyright Fertility Institute of the Mid-South, Inc. Web Version C. 2020. www.danmartinmd.com/files/lae1990.pdf

Citations

Did You Know?

9. Bao C, Wang H, Fang H. Genomic Evidence Supports the Recognition of Endometriosis as an Inflammatory Systemic Disease and Reveals Disease=Specific Therapeutic Potentials of Targeting Neutrophil Degranulation. Front Immunol.2022;13: article 758440.Doi:10.3389/fimmu.2022.758440

10. Endometriosis (Fact Page). Autoimmune Diseases List. Global Autoimmune Institute. https://www.autoimmuneinstitute.org (accessed February 4, 2024).

11. Lamceva J, Uljanovs R, Strumfa I. The Main Theories on the Pathogenesis of Endometriosis. Int'l J Mol Science.2023; 24:4254. Doi: 10.3990/ijms24054254

12. Tabibian N, Swehli E, Boyd A, Umbreen A, Tabibian JH. Abdominal adhesions: A practical review of an often overlooked entity. Ann Med Surg (Lond).2017;15:9. Doi:10.1016.j.amsu.2017.01.021

Citations

Did You Know?

13. Imudia A, Kumar S, Saed G, Diamond M. Pathogenesis, Intraabdominal and Pelvic Adhesion Development. Sem Repro Med. 2008;26(4):289-2997. Doi: 10.1055/s-0028-1082387

14. Abd El-Kader AI, Goried AS, Mohammed H, Lofty Mohammed S. Impact of Endometriosis-Related Adhesions on Quality of Life Among Infertile Women. Int J Fert Steril.2019;13(1): 72-6. Doi: 10.22074/ijfs.2019.5572

15. Smalarz B, Szyllok K, Romanowicz H. Endometriosis: Epidemiology, Classification, Pathogenesis, Treatment and Genetics. Review of Literature. Int'l J Mol Sci.2021; 22:10554. Doi: 10.3390/ijms221910554

16. Zondervan KT, Becker CM, Missmer SA. Endometriosis. N Engl J Med. 2020;382:1244-56.

Citations

Did You Know?

17. Shim JY, Laufer MR, Grimstad FW. Dysmenorrhea and Endometriosis in Transgender Adolescents. J Pediatr Adolesc Gynecol.2020;33(5):524-528. Doi: 10.1016/j.jpag.2020.06.001

18. Balgobind S, Menon VA, McKenzie P, Gupta R, Canagasingham B, O'Toole S. The bleeding obvious: A case of male endometriosis. Pathology.2019;51(S1);pp.S71–141.

19. March E, Laufer MR. Endometriosis in premenarchial girls without an associated obstructive anomaly. Fert Stert..2005;83: pp. 758-760.

20. Tronkon JK, et al. Endometriosis in a patient with Mayer-Rokitansky-Kuster-Hauser syndrome. Case Rep Obstet Gynecol. 2014;2014:376231. Doi: 10.1155/2014/376231

21. Rizk B. Recurrence of endometriosis after hysterectomy. Facts Views Vis. Obgyn. 2014;6(4):219-27.

Citations

Did You Know?

22. Haas D, et al. Endometriosis: a premenopausal disease? Age pattern in 42,079 patients with endometriosis. Arch Gynecol Obstet.2012;286: 667–670. DOI 10.1007/s00404-012-2361-z

23. Morotti M, et al. Endometriosis in menopause: a single institution experience. Arch Gynecol Obstet .2021; 286(6):1571-5. Doi: 10.1007/s00404-012-2473-5

24. Baldi A, et al. logical and Immunohistochemical Characterization of a Case of Endometriosis in a Guinea Pig (Cavia schudi). Case Reports in Veterinary Medicine. 2017. Doi: 10.1155/2017/4594510

25. Paiva BHA, et al. A rare case of endometrioma in a bitch Acta Veterinari. Scandinavica.2015.57:31. Doi: 10.101186/s13028-015-0123-1

26. Human and Primates estrus vs anestrus Demirel MA. A Case of Spontaneous Abortion Related to Ovarian Endometriosis in a Golden Retriever Dog. Iranian J Veterinarian Research. 2017;18(1):63-66.

Citations
Did You Know?

27. Mason-Jones AJ, Woodward A, Fryer J. Understanding diagnostic delay for endometriosis: a scoping review. https://www.medrxiv.org/content/10.1101/2024.01.08.24300988v1.full.pdf. (prepublication)

28. "What does endometriosis feel like?" www.endocenter.org/do-you-have -endo/ (accessed January 30,2024).

29. Smalarz B, Szyllok K, Romanowicz H. Endometriosis: Epidemiology, Classification, Pathologenesis, Treatment and Genetics. Review of Literature. Intl J Mol Sci. 2021;22:10554. Doi: 10.3390/ijms221910554

30. DiBenedetti D, Soliman A, Gupta C, Surrey ES. Patient's perspectives of endometriosis- related fatigue: qualitative interviews. J Patient Rep Outcomes.2020; 4:33. Doi 10.1186/s41687-020-00200-1

Citations
Did You Know?

31. Boneva RS, Lin Js, Wiesser F, Nater UM, Ditzen B, Taylor RN, Unger ER. Endometriosis as a Comorbid Condition in Chronic Fatigue Syndrome (CFS): Secondary Analysis of Data From a CFS Case Control Study. Front Pediatr 2019;7:195. Doi: 10.3389/fped.2019.00195

32. Shafrir AL, Palmor MC, Fourquet J, DiVasta AD, Farland LV et al. Co-occurrence of immune-mediated conditions and endometriosis among adolescents and adult women. Am J Reprod Immunol. 2021;86(1); e13404. Doi: 10.1111/aji.13404

33. Chiaffarino F, et al. Endometriosis and irritable bowel syndrome: a systematic review and meta- analysis. Archives Gynec Obstet.(2020). Dio:10/1007/s/00404-020-05797-8

34. DiVasta AD, et al. Overlap between irritable bowel syndrome diagnosis and endometriosis in adolescents. Clinical Gastroenterology and Hepatology. 2020.

Citations
Did You Know?

35. Miller JA, et al. The prevalence of migraines in adolescents with endometriosis. Fert Stert 2017. Doi.org/10.1016/j.fertnstert.2017.12.016

36. Shim JY, Laufer MR. Adolescent Endometriosis: an Update. J Pediatric Adolesc Gynec. 2020. Doi: 10.1016/j.jpag.2019.11.011

37. Al-Shaiji TF, Alshammaa DH,Al-Mansouri MM, Al-Terkj A. Association of endometriosis with Interstitial Cystitis in Chronic Pelvic Pain Syndrome: Short Narrative on Prevalence, Diagnostic Limitations and Clinical Implications. Qatar Med J.2021;3:50.

38. Shafrir AL, Palmor MC, Fourquet J, DiVasta AD, Farland LV et al. Co-occurrence of immune-mediated conditions and endometriosis among adolescents and adult women. Am J Reprod.2021;86(1):313404. Doi: 10.1111.aji.13404

Citations
Did You Know?

39. Rahmioglue N et al. The genetic basis of endometriosis and comorbidity with other pain and inflammatory conditions. Nat Genet.2023; 55(3):423-436. Doi: 10.1038/s41588-023-01323-z

40. Wirth KJ, Lohn M. Myalgic Encephalomyelitis/Chronic Fatigue Syndrome (ME/CFS) and Comorbidities: Linked by Vascular Pathomechanisms and Vasoactive Mediators? Medicina.2023;59:978. Doi:10.3390/medicina59050978

41. Vazgiourakis VM, Zervou M, Papageorgiou L, Spandidos DA, Vlachakis D et al. Association of endometriosis with cardiovascular disease: Genetic aspects (Review). Int'l J Mol Med. 2023;1:29. Doi: 10.3892/ijmm.2023.5232

42. Shigesi N, Kvaskoff M, Kirtley S, Feng Q, Fang H et al. The association between endometriosis and autoimmune diseases: a systematic review and meta-analysis. Hum Reprod Update.2019;25(4):486-503. Doi: 10.1093/humupd/dmz014

Citations

Did You Know?

43. Porpora MG, Scaramuzzino S, Sangiuliano C, Piacenti I, Ostuni R et al. High Prevalence of autoimmune diseases in women with endometriosis: a case-control study. Gynecol Endocrinol.2020;36(4):356-359. Doi: 10.1080/09513590.2019.1655727

44. Ruffo G, Scopelliti F, Manzoni A, Sartori A, Rossini R et al. Long-Term Outcomes after Resections for Deep infiltrating Endometriosis: A Single-Center Experience after 900 Cases. Biomed Res Int'l (2014).

45. Matalliotakis M, Goulielmos GNB, Kalogiannidis I, Koumantakis G, Matalliotakis L et al. al. Extra pelvic endometriosis: Epidemiologic analysis on 200 cases from two different countries. Eur J Obstet Gynec Repro Bio. Doi:10.1016/j.ejogrb.2017.08.019

46. Chamie LP, et al. Atypical sites of deeply infiltrative endometriosis: clinical characteristics and imaging findings. Radiographics 2018 Vol 38;pp 309-328. Doi: 10.1148/rg.2018170093.

Citations
Did You Know?

47. Lukac S, Schmid M, Pfister K, Janni W, Schäffler H, Dayan D: Extragenital endometriosis in the differential diagnosis of non-gynecological diseases. Dtsch Arztebl Int.2022; 119: 361–7. DOI: 10.3238/arztebl.m2022.0176

48. Charatsi D, Koukkoura O, Ntavela IG, Hintziou F, Gkorila G et al. Gastrointestinal and Urinary Tract Endometriosis: A Review on the Commonest Locations of Extrapelvic Endometriosis. Adv Med.2018;3461209. Doi: 10.1155/2018/3461209

49. Huang QF, Jiang B, Yang X, Yu B, Hu XP. Primary versus secondary cutaneous endometriosis: Literature review and case study. Heliyon. 2023 Sep 26;9(10):e20094. Doi: 10.1016/j.heliyon.2023.e20094

50. "Symptoms of Hepatic Endometriosis" https://extrapelvicnotrare.org/liver-hepatic-endometriosis/ (accessed Feb. 4, 2024).

Citations

Did You Know?

51. Pancreatic Endometriosis. https://extrapelvicnotrare.org/pancreatic-endometriosis/ (accessed Feb 4, 2024).

52. ASRM. Practice Committee of the American Society for Reproductive Medicine Endometriosis and infertility: a committee opinion. Fertil Steril. 2012;98:591–598. Doi: 10.1016/j.fertnstert.2012.05.031

53. Chen LH, Lo, WC, Huan HY, Wu HS. A Lifelong Impact on Endometriosis: Pathophysiology and Pharmacological Treatment. Int J Mol Sci.2023;24(8):7503.Doi: 10.3390/ijms24087503

54. Ostiz LM et al. Cyclic hematochezia in a young woman with appendiceal endometriosis. Rev Esp Enferm Dig.2024.116(1):37038. Doi: 10.17235/reed.2022.9257/2022

55. Quintana-Rapatalo RJ, Phrathep DD, Ward I, Healey KD, Anthony S, Herman M. Cecal Endometriosis Presenting as Hematochezia in a Postmenopausal Female. Cureus. 2023;17;15(1):e33886. Doi: 10.7759/cureus.33886

Citations
Did You Know?

56. Arjonilla M, Khander A, Pal T, Jamorabo D. Intestinal Endometriosis Leading to Recurrent Hematochezia. ACG Case Rep J. 2022;9(10): e00872. Doi: 10.14309/crj.0000000000000872

57. Aldhaheri S, Suarthana E, Capmas P, Badeghiesh A, Gil Y, Tulandi T. Association Between Bowel Obstruction or Intussusception and Endometriosis. J Obstet Gynaecol Can. 2021;43(4): 440-446. Doi: 10.1016/j.jogc.2020.12.008

58. Galazis N, Arul D, Wilson J, Pisal N. Bowel endometriosis. BMJ Case Rep. 2014 10;2014: bcr2013202140. Doi: 10.1136/bcr-2013-202140

59. Kobayashi K, Yamadera M,Takeo H, Murayama M. Small bowel obstruction caused by appendiceal and ileal endometriosis: a case report. J Surg Case Rep.2022;2022(6):rjac282. Doi: 10.1093/jscr/rjac282

Citations
Did You Know?

60. Bray-Beraldo F, Pellino G, Ribeiro MAF Jr, Pereira AMG, Lopes RGC, Mabrouk M, Di Saverio Evaluation of Bowel Function After Surgical Treatment for Intestinal Endometriosis: A Prospective Study. Dis Colon Rectum. 2021;64(10):1267-1275. Doi: 10.1097/DCR.0000000000001890

61. Dior UP, Reddington C, Cheng C, Levin G, Mc Inerney C, Moss A, Healey M. Lower gastrointestinal function after surgery for deep endometriosis: A prospective cohort study. Int J Gynaecol Obstet. 2023;160(1): 280-288. Doi: 10.1002/ijgo.14350

62. Peng C, Zhang DY, Zhou YF, Huang Y, Lu Y, Xue Q. [Clinical analysis of ureteral endometriosis complicated with hydronephrosis: 92 cases series]. Zhonghua Fu Chan Ke Za Zhi.2021;56(12) :836-841. Chinese. Doi: 10.3760/cma.j.cn112141-20210803-00418

Citations

Did You Know?

63. Yang K, Cheng S, Cai Y, Qiao J, Xu Y, Li X, Xiong S, Lu Y, Mei A, Li X, Zhou L. Clinical characteristics and surgical treatment of ureteral endometriosis: our experience with 40 cases. BMC Womens Health. 2021;21(1):206. Doi: 10.1186/s12905-021-01349-7

64. Sherman AK, MacLachlan LS. A Review of Urinary Tract Endometriosis. Curr Urol Rep. 2022;23(10):219-223. Doi: 10.1007/s11934-022-01107-8

65. Gabriel I, Vitonis AF, Missmer SA, Fadayomi A, DiVasta AD, Terry KL, Minassian VA. Association between endometriosis and lower urinary tract symptoms. Fertil Steril. 2022 Apr;117(4):822-830. Doi:10.1016/j.fertnstert.2022.01.003

66. Froc E, Dubernard G, Bendifallah S, Hermouet E, Rubod-Dit-Guillet C, Canis M, Warembourg S, Golfier F, Fauconnier A, Roman H, Philip CA. Clinical characteristics of urinary tract endometriosis: A one-year national series of 232 patients from 31 endometriosis (cont)

Citations
Did You Know?

66. (cont) expert centers (by the FRIENDS group). Eur J Obstet Gynecol Reprod Biol.2021;264: 155-161. Doi: 10.1016/j.ejogrb.2021.06.018

67. Fournel L, Bobbio A, Robin E, Canny-Hamelin E, Alifano M, Regnard JF. Clinical presentation and treatment of catamenial pneumothorax and endometriosis-related pneumothorax. Expert Rev Respir Med. 2018 Dec;12(12):1031-1036. Doi: 10.1080/17476348.2018.1551133

68. Yukumi S, Suzuki H, Morimoto M, Shigematsu H, Sugimoto R, Sakao N, Abe M, Watanabe A, Kitazawa S, Sano Y. A case of thoracic endometriosis-related pneumothorax in a menopausal woman. Gen Thorac Cardiovasc Surg. 2020;68(12): 1584-1586. Doi: 10.1007/s11748-020-01381-8

69. Yukumi S, Suzuki H, Morimoto M, Shigematsu H, Okazaki M, Abe M, Kitazawa S, Nakamura K, Sano Y. Two Young Women with Left-sided Pneumothorax Due to Thoracic Endometriosis.Intern Med. 2016;55(23): (cont)

Citations
Did You Know?

69. Yukumi S et al. (cont) 3491-3493. Doi:10.2169/internalmedicine.55.7187

70. Inoue T, Chida M, Inaba H, Tamura M, Kobayashi S, Sado T. Juvenile catamenial pneumothorax: institutional report and review. J Cardiothorac Surg. 2015;10:83. Doi: 10.1186/s13019-015-0289-7

71. Ciriaco P, Muriana P, Lembo R, Carretta A, Negri G. Treatment of Thoracic Endometriosis Syndrome: A Meta-Analysis and Review. Ann Thorac Surg. 2022;113(1): 324-336. Doi: 10.1016/j.athoracsur.2020.09.064

72. Bobbio A, Canny E, Mansuet Lupo A, Lococo F, Legras A, Magdeleinat P, Regnard JF, Gompel A, Damotte D, Alifano M. Thoracic Endometriosis Syndrome Other Than Pneumothorax: Clinical and Pathological Findings. Ann Thorac Surg. 2017;104(6):1865-1871. Doi: 10.1016/j.athoracsur.2017.06.

Citations
Did You Know?

73. Porcel JM, Sancho-Marquina P, Monteagudo P, Bielsa S. Pleural effusion secondary to endometriosis: A systematic review. Am J Med Sci. 2023;366(4):296-304. Doi: 10.1016/j.amjms.2023.08.003

74. Chetambath R, Kumar P, Nandini V, Chandran S, Chacko A. Catamenial haemothorax-A rare cause of pleural effusion. Lung India. 2023;40(6):541-544. Doi: 10.4103/lungindia.lungindia_144_23

75. Dai Y, Li MH, Liu YJ, Liu B, Wu YS, Lang JH, Zhang ZY, Leng JH. Thoracic endometriosis presented as catamenial hemoptysis: a case series of a rare disease.Cur Med Res Opin. 2021;37(4):685-691. Doi: 10.1080/03007995.2021.1885363

76. Bala A, Salim RA, Deliwala S, Obeid M, Bachuwa G. Cyclical Hemoptysis and Pelvic Pain in a Young Female: A Sign of Thoracic Endometriosis Syndrome. Cureus. 2020;12(10):e11078. Doi: 10.7759/cureus.11078

Citations
Did You Know?

77. Roman H, Dehan L, Merlot B, Berby B, Forestier D, Seyer-Hansen M, Abo C, Tuech JJ. Postoperative Outcomes after Surgery for Deep Endometriosis of the Sacral Plexus and Sciatic Nerve: A 52-patient Consecutive Series. JMIG.2021;28(7):1375-1383. Doi: 10.1016/j.jmig.2020.10.018

78. Possover M. Laparoscopic morphological aspects and tentative explanation of the aetiopathogenesis of isolated endometriosis of the sciatic nerve: a review based on 267 patients. Facts Views Vis Obgyn. 2021;13(4): 369-375. Doi: 10.52054/FVVO.13.4.047

Citations
A to Z

Adductors (muscle group)
Fabrini M. Large-muscle endometriosis involving the adductor tight compartment: case report. JMIG.2010;17(2):258-261.

Adrenal Gland
Rehman J et al. A case of successful laparoscopic resection of adrenal gland endometriosis. Fert Ster.2008;90(05):2015. e7-e9.

Alcock's Canal
Nehme-Schuster H, et al. Alcock's canal syndrome revealing endometriosis. Lancet.2005;366:1238.

Alveoli
Takahashi R et al. Left-sided catamenial pneumothorax with thoracic endometriosis and bullae in the alveolar wall. Ann Thorac Cardiovasc Surg.2017;23:108-112.

Aorta
Notzold A et al. Endometriosis in the thoracic aorta. NEJM.2018;339(114):1002-1003.

Citations
A to Z

Appendix
Lebastchi A et al. Appendiceal endometriosis in a pregnant woman presenting with acute perforated appendicitis. J Surg Case Rep.2013;3(12):104.

Ascending Colon
Horsley-Silva, J; Roque, MV. Colonic Endometriosis: A Case of Chronic Abdominal Pain. American J of Gastroenterology. 2012;107:S477-S478.

Biceps Femoris (muscle)
Giangarra C et al. Endometriosis in the biceps femoris: A case report and review of the literature. J Bone Jt Surgery. 1987;69(2):290-292.

Bladder
Gabriel B et al. Prevalence and management of urinary tract endometriosis: a clinical case series. Urology.2011;78(6):1269-74.

Bone
Redwine DB, Sharpe DR. Endometriosis of the obturator nerve. A case report. J Reprod Med. 1990;35(4):434-5 (abstract).

Citations
A to Z

Brachioradialis (muscle)
Navratil E, Kramer A.Klin. Wschr. 1936;15.

Breast
Al-wageeh S et al. Ectopic endometriosis presenting as a breast abscess in a teenager. J Pediatric Surg Case Rep.2021.75;102073. Doi.org/10.1016/j.epse.2021.102073.

McArthur GJ,. Lowndes S, Meagher PS. Endometriosis following free DIEP breast reconstruction. JPRAS. 2009.63(3):420-1.

Bronchiolie(s)
Kuo PH et al. Bronchoscopic and angiographic findings in tracehobronchial endometriosis. Thorax.1996;51:1050-1.

Cecum
Rivkine E et al. Ileocolic intussusception due to a cecal endometriosis: case report and review of literature. Diagnostic Pathology.2012;2;7:62.

Cerebellum
Sarma D et al. Cerebellar Endometriosis. AJR.June 2004; 182:1543-46.

Citations
A to Z

Cerebrum
Thibodeau L et al. Cerebral endometriosis. J Neurosurg. April 1987;66:609-610.

Common Bile Duct
Chien-Chu L, Jiann-Ming Wu. Endometriosis of the Common Bile Duct. J Gastrointest Surg.2023;27(8):1749-1750. Doi: 10.1007/s11605-023-05658-0

Conus Medullaris
Agrawal A et al. Intramedullary endometriosis of the conus medullaris: case report. Neurosurgery. Aug 2006.59;(2):E427-8.

Deltoid Muscle
Aron SE. Endomertriosis in the region of the deltoid muscle. Arkhiv Patologii.1957;19(7):67-8 (russian).

Nagamoto Y et al. Endometriosis in the deltoid muscle: a case report. Eur J Orhop Surg Traumatol.2012;22:497-500.

Citations
A to Z

Deltoid Muscle (cont)
Wang J et al. Endometriosis of extra-abdominal soft tissues: A tertiary center experience. Int'l J Surg Path. 2016. Doi:10.1177/1066896916644322

Descending Colon
Ihyun K, Min-Jeong K, Hong Il H, Kwanseop L, Soo Kee M. Descending Colon Endometriosis Misdiagnosed as Diverticulitis. J of the Korean Society of Radiology 2016; 75(3): 203-207. Doi.org/10.3348/jksr.2016.75.3.203

Diaphragm
Channabasavaiah AD, Joseph JV. Thoracic endometriosis: revisiting the association between clinical presentation and thoracic pathology based on thoracoscopic findings in 110 patients.Medicine.2010;89(3):183-8.

Nezhat C et al. Laparoscopic management of diaphragm endometriosis: report of two cases and review of the literature.JMIG.2005;12:196-20

Citations
A to Z

Duodenum
Piccinnni G, Massimiliano De Luca G, Lafranceschina S et al. Laparoscopic Treatment of a Retroduodenopancreatic Endometriotic Cyst Observed Postpartum. J Laparoendoscopic & Adv Surg Tech. 2016. DOI: 10.1089/lap.2016.0319

Epididymis
Giannarini G et al. Cystic Endometriosis of the Epididymis. Urology.2006;68:203.e1-203.e3.

External Iliac Vein
Zamurovic M. Rare extrapelvic endometriosis on iliac vein wall-Diagnosis and treatment. Clin Exp Obstet Gynecol. 2014;41(3):349-350 (abstract).

External Oblique (muscle)
Chiaramonte R et al. Thrombosis of iliac vessels, a rare complication of endometriosis: Case report and review of literature. J Adv Res.2017;8:1-5.

Eyelid
Sharghik G et al. Endometriosis of the eyelid, an extraabdominal location highlighting the spectrum of disease. Am J Dermatopathol. 2019;41(8):593-5.

Citations
A to Z

Falciform Ligament

Surgical images.arizona.edu/medical-image-vocabulary/endometriosis-umbilicus-and-falciform-ligament (accessed 07/06/2022).

Femoral Nerve

Andrade C et al. Laparoscopic neurolysis of deep endometriosis Infiltrating left femoral nerve: Case report. Surg Technol Int.2015;27:163-8 (abstract).

Niro J et al. Endometriotic lesions of the lower troncular nerves.Gynecol Obstet Fertil.2014; 42(10):702-5.

Femoral Vein

Recalde Al, Majmudar B. Endometriosis involving the femoral vein. South Med J.1977;70(1):69-74.

Femur

Oei SC et al. Aggressive Endometriosis in bone. Lancet.1992;339:1477-8.

Fingertip

Saubhagya Kumar Jena et al. Spontaneous fingertip endometriosis: A rare case report. J Clin Diag Res. 2015;9(5):Q101.

Citations
A to Z

Gallbladder
Iafrate F et al. Gallbladder and muscular endometriosis: A case report. Abdom Imaging. 2013;38(1):120-4.

Saldona DG et al. Gallbladder endometrioma associated with obstructive jaundice and a serous ovarian cystic adenoma.
South Med J.2010.103: 1250-2.

Gastrocnemius (muscle)
Omero Benedictor Poli-Neto et al. Endometriosis of the soleus and gastrocnemius muscles.
Fert Ster. 2009;91(4)1294.e14.

Gluteus Medius and Maximus (muscles)
Botha AJ et al. Endometriosis in gluteal muscle with surgical implantation. Acta Orthopaedica Scandinavica.1991;62(5):497-9.

Guida M et al. Isolated extrapelvic endometriosis of the gluteal muscle. JMIG.2008;16(1):95-97.

Citations
A to Z

Groin
Yi Ding et al. Endometriosis mimicking soft-tissue neoplasm: A potential diagnostic pitfall. Cancer Control. 2017;24(1):83-8.

Heart
Felson H et al. Stromal endometriosis involving the heart. Amer J Med. Dec 1960;1072-6.

Ileum
Bratu D et al. A rare case of ileus caused by ileum endometriosis. Int'l J Surgical Case Rep.2016;26:24-6.

Ileocecal Valve
Cirillo F et al. Endometriosis of the caecum and ileo-caecal valve. A case report and review of the literature. Chiro Ital. 2008;60(4):603-6.

Mizuta N et al. Bowel endometriosis treated with simultaneous ileocecal and rectal section. J Surg Case Rep. 2018;2:1-4.

Citations
A to Z

Ileocecal Valve (cont)
Podgaec S et al. Epigastric pain relating to menses can be a symptom of bowel endometriosis. Sao Paulo Med J. 2008;126(4): 242-4.

Ilioinguinal Nerve
Pelligrini V et al. Endometrioma of the Pubis: A differential diagnosis of hip pain. J Bone Jt Surgery Am.1981;63(8):1333-4.

Inferior Vena Cava
Post menopause endometriosis with inferior vena cava invasion requiring surgical management. Human Repro. 2011;26(10):2709-12.

Inguinal Ligament & Canal
Kim DH et al. Inguinal endometriosis in a patient without a previous history of gynecological surgery. Obstet Gynecol Sci.2014;57(2):172-5.

Ischiorectal Fossa
Ramalingappa A, Reddy Yashoda. A rare presentation of endometriosis. J Obstet Gyn India. 2012;62(S1):S94-6.

Citations
A to Z

Jejunum

Berjemann W, Heuer C. Extragenital endometriosis with multiple stenosis of the small intestine. Fortschr Med. 1992;110(15):281-4.

Kidney

Jie Yang et al. Renal endometriosis tends to be misdiagnosed as renal tumor: A rare case report. Int'l Surg.2015;100:376-80.

Bazoz-Malik G et al. Endometrioma of the kidney: Case report. J Urology. 1979;123:422-3.

Giambelluca D et al. Renal endometriosis mimicking complicated cysts of kidney: report of two cases. G Chiro.2017;38(5):250-5.

Bailey AP et al. Florid endometriosis in a postmenopausal woman. Fert Ster.2010;94(7): 2769e1-4.

Knee

Patel VC et al. Endometriosis at the knee. A case report. Clin Orthop Relat Res.1982;Nov-Dec 171:140-4.

Citations
A to Z

Lip

Laurent WCP, Gerard EBJ, Stive TF, Gochede G, Charles EM. (2024) Oral Endometriosis: An Unexpected Presentation of An Exceptional Pathology. J Oral Med and Dent Res. 5(4):1-6. Doi:10.52793/JOMDR.2024.5(4)-71

Liver

Nezhat C et al. Laparoscopic management of hepatic endometriosis: report of two cases and review of the literature. JMIG.2005;12:196-200.

Lymph Node

Li et al. Endometriosis in para-aortic lymph node resembling a malignancy: a case report and literature review. BMC Women's Health (2022) 22:101 https://doi.org/10.1186/s12905-022-01659-4

Mandible

Contreras Gala KL, Villafuerte Roza M. Jaw Region Endometriosis: Case Report. Rev Fac Med Hum 2011;21(4)"889-895. Doi: 10.25176/RFMH.v2114.4033

Citations
A to Z

Mediastinum
Pichyurov AA, et al. Thoracic endometriosis: the rare pathology in thoracic surgery. Vestnik Khirurgiimen I.I. Grekova (abstract English). Jan 2014.173(1):26-9.

Mesentery
Bailey AP et al.Florid endometriosis in a postmenopausal woman. Fert Stert.2010;94(7): 2769e1-4.

Nerve Root
Lemos et al. Sacral nerve infiltrative endometriosis presenting as perimenstrual right-sided sciatica and bladder atonia: case report and description of surgical technique. JMIG.2012;19(3): 396-400.

Nose (nasal mucosa)
Mignemi G. et al. A case report of nasal endometriosis in a patient affected by Behcet's Disease.JMIG.2012;19:514-16.

Laghzaoui M, Laghzaoui O. Endometriose nasale: a propos d'un cas. J Gynecol Obstet Biol Reprod. 2001; 30(8):786-8.

Citations
A to Z

Obturator Internus (muscle)
Baskar O, Ozdemir F. Endometriosis of the sciatic nerve with cyclical sciatica. Acta Media Lituanca.2012;21(3):99-102.

Obturator Nerve
Redwine DB, Sharpe DR. Endometriosis of the obturator nerve. J Reprod Med.1990;35:434-5.

Ekpo G et al. Laparoscopic excision of endometriosis of the obturator nerve: a case report.JMIG.2007;14(6):746-6.

Omentum
Rorat E, Wallach RC. Endometriosis of the omentum and borderline ovarian malignancy. Eur J Gynaecol Oncol. 1986:7(1).

Pardeep Athwal et al. A case of multisystem endometriosis. Gen Radiology.2013;7(10):1-6.

Pancreas
Lee DS et al. A case of pancreatic endometrial cyst. Korean J of Int Med.2002;17(4):266-9.

Citations
A to Z

Parietal Pleura
Channabasavaich AD, Joseph JV. Thoracic endometriosis: Revisiting the association between clinical presentation and thoracic pathology based on thoracoscopic findings in 110 patients. Medicine.2010;89(3):83-8.

Perianal
McComb K, Barghash M, Eltyef S. Perianal endometriosis: An uncommon site for a common problem. Cureus. 2023;15(9):e44840.

Pericardium
Ceccaroni M et al. Pericardial, pleural and diaphragmatic endometriosis in association with pelvic peritoneal and bowel endometriosis: a case report and review of the literature. Video surgery and other mini-invasive tech. 2012;7(2):122-7.

Piriformis (muscle)
Dominguez-Poez M et al. Sciatica secondary to extrapelvic endometriosis affecting the piriformis muscle. Case report. Neurocirugia.2012;23(4): 170-2.

Citations
A to Z

Pronator Teres (muscle)
Smith KL, He L, Adhya J, Ercolano L. Intramuscular endometriosis of the forearm: a case report. Skeletal Radiology (2024) 53:2735-2740. Doi: 10.1007/s00256-024-04648

Prostate
Beckman EN et al. Endometriosis of the Prostate. Amer J Surg Pathol. 1985;9(5):374-379.

Psoas Major (muscle)
Bhat SN et al. Endometriosis presenting like a psoas abscess. Saudi Med J.2007;28(6):952-4 (abstract).

Pyramidalis (muscle)
Crespo R et al. Pyrimidalis muscle endometriosis in absence of previous surgery. Int'l J Gynaecol Obstet.2005;89(2):148-9 (abstract).

Perineum
Li J et al. Diagnosis and treatment of perineal endometriosis: review of 17 cases. Arch Gynecol Obstet .2015;292(6):1295-9.

Citations A to Z

Quadriceps (muscle group)
Pareja LA et al. Malignant endometrioma in the lower left limb. Cir Esp.2018;96(3):173-80.

Cauda EQuina
Agrawal et al. Intramedullary endometriosis of the conus medullaris: case report. Neurosurgery.2006; 59(2):E427-8.

De Sousa et al. Neural involvement in endometriosis: review of anatomic distribution and mechanisms. Clin Anat.2015;28(8):1029-30.

Rectum
Mizuta N et al. Bowel endometriosis treated with simultaneous ileocecal and rectal resection. J Surg Case Reports.2018;2:1-4.

Rectus Abdominus (muscle)
Endometriosis externa within the rectus abdominus muscle. Unusual Cer Derg.2014;30: 165-8.

Rectus Femoris (muscle)
Pareja LA et al. Endometrioma malignizada localizadoe en el miembro inferior. Cir Esp.2018; 96:173-4.

Citations
A to Z

Round Ligament
Khetan N et al. Endometriosis: presentation to general surgeons. Ann R Coll Surg Engl.1999;81: 255-9

Scar and Skin
Tsenov D. Endometriosis in the surgical scar from cesarean section. Akush Ginekol.2000;39(1):50-1.

Ecker A et al. Abdominal wall endometriosis: a 12-year experience at a large academic institution.JMIG.2014;S31.

Sciatic Nerve
Possover M. Five-year follow-up after laparoscopic large nerve resection for deep infiltrating sciatic nerve endometriosis. JMIG.2017;24(5):822-6.

Capek S et al. Sequential imaging of intraneural sciatic nerve endometriosis provides insights into symptoms of cyclical sciatica. Acta Neurochir. 2016;158(3):507-12.

Citations
A to Z

Sciatic Nerve (cont)
Baskan O, Ozdemir F. Endometriosis of the sciatic nerve with cyclic sciatica. Acta Medica Lituanica.2014;21(3):99-102.

Semitendinosus + Semimembranosus (muscles)
Schlicke CP Lt. Col. Ectopic endometrial tissue of the thigh. JAMA.1947;122(8):445-6.

Sigmoid Colon
Dimoulios P et al. A case of sigmoid endometriosis difficult to differentiate from colon cancer. BMC Gastroenterology. 2003;3:18.

Soleus (muscle)
Omero Benedictor Poli-Neto et al. Endometriosis of the soleus and gastrocnemius muscles. Fert Stert.2009;91(4): 1294.e14.

Saberi S et al. Endometriosis: A case report and review of the musculoskeletal involvement. Am J Orthop.2009;38(11):E175-178.

Soleus muscle
Poli-Neto et al. Endometriosis of the Soleus and Gastrocnemius muscles. Fert Stert.2009;91(4): 1294e.13-15.

Citations
A to Z

Spleen

Weyl W et al. Splenic lesion mimicking breast metastasis: The first description of the splenic parenchymal endometriosis.JEPPD.2020. Doi: 10.1177/2284026520960846

Stomach

Jong Kum Ho et al. An extremely rare case of gastric subepithelial tumor: gastric endometriosis. Clin Endoscopy. 2015;48:74-77.

Subarachnoid Space

Lombardo L et al. Subarchnoid haemorhage due to endometriosis of the spinal cord. Neurology. 1968;18:423-6.

Superior Gluteal Nerve

Reddy S et al. Endometriosis of the Superior Gluteal Nerve. Skeletal Radiology.2007;36(9): 879-883.

Testicle

Al-Obaidy KI, Icrees MT. Endometriosis with Cystic Degeneration: A Rare Disease of Males. Int'l J Surg Pathol.2018.orcide.org/0000-0001-9890-8751.

Citations
A to Z

Testicle
Draeger DL et al. Paratesticular Multicystic Tumor of the Tunica VaginalisTestis as Rare Paratesticular Cystadenoma. Urologia Int'l. DOI: 10.1159/000458159

Fukunaga M. Paratesticular Endometriosis in a Man with Prolonged Hormone Therapy for Prostate Carcinoma. Pathology- Research and practice.2012;208:59-61.

Young RH, Robert SE. Testicular and Paratesticular Tumors and Tumor-Like Lesions of Ovarian Common Epithelial and Mullerian Types. Am J Clin Pathol.1986;86:146-152.

Thumb
Das Gupta S et al. Endometriosis in the thumb. J Indian Med Assoc.1985;83(4):122-123.

Trachea (windpipe)
Kuo PH et al. Bronchoscopic and angiographic findings in tracheobronchial endometriosis. Thorax.1996.51:1050.

Citations
A to Z

Transverse Colon
Hartmann D. et al. Endometriose des Colon transversum. Dtsch Med Wochenschr.2002;127:237-2320.

Trapezius (muscle)
Gennari and Luciani. Un coso di endometriosi de musculo Trapezio. Ricevuto in Redozione. 1965: 361-66. (Italian). A case of endometriosis of the trapezius muscle. Tumol.1965; 51:36366.

Umbilicus (belly button)
Ecker A et al. Abdominal wall endometriosis: a 12-year experience at a large academic institution. JMIG.2014:S31.

Ureter
Ping W et al. Hydronephrosis due to ureteral endometriosis in women of reproductive age. Int'l J Clin Exp Med.2015;8(1): 1059-65.

Bailey AP et al. Florid endometriosis in a postmenopausal woman. Fert Stert.2010;94(7): 2769e.1-4.

Citations
A to Z

Urethra

Chowdy AA et al. Endometriosis presenting as a urethral diverticulum: a case report. J Reprod Med.2004;49(4):321-3.

Vagina

Nelson P. Endometriosis presenting as a vaginal mass. Case Reports.2018;23.

Vas Deferens

Rei C et al. Endometriosis in a Man as a Rare Source of Abdominal Pain: A Case Report and Review of the Literature. Case Rep Obstet Gynecol. Elsevier. (2018). DOI:10.1155/2018/2083121

Vertebra

Dongxu Z et al. Low back pain tied to spinal endometriosis. Eur Spine J. 2014;23(suppl2):214-7.

Visceral Pleura

Channabasovaiah AD, Joseph JV. Thoracic endometriosis: revisiting the association between clinical presentation and thoracic pathology based on thoracoscopic findings in 110 patients. Medicine.2010; 89(3):183-8.

Citations
A to Z

Visceral Pleura (cont)
Takahashi R et al. Left-sided catamenial pneumothorax with thoracic endometriosis and bullae in the alveolar wall. Ann Thorac Cardiovasc Surg.2017;23:108-11.

Vulva
Brug P et al. Vulvar endometriosis presenting with dyspareunia: a case report. J Reprod Med. 2012;57(3-4):75-7.

Wrist
Ding Y et al. Endometriosis mimicking soft tissue neoplasms: a potential diagnostic pitfall. Cancer Control. 2017;24(1):83-8.

Sacral PleXus
Possover M et al. Laparoscopic therapy for endometriosis and vascular entrapment of sacral plexus. Fert Stert.2011; 95(2):756-8 (abstract).

ParenchYma (lung + liver)
Fang H et al. Catamenial pneumothorax due to bilateral pulmonary endometriosis. Respir Care.2012;57(7):1182-5.

Citations
A to Z

ParenchYma (kidney, liver, lung, pancreas, spleen, stomach). Poh CL et al. Pulmonary parenchymal endometriosis presenting as bilateral pneumothorax. J Obstet Gynaec. 2011;31(5):452-8.

Other locations include

- kidney
- liver
- lung
- pancreas
- spleen
- stomach

Z-Lines

Definition: Z-filament is the thin zigzag strand at the Z-Line of striated muscle (skeletal). The Z-line is attachment site for contractile filament (actin).

Example locations include:

- Adductors (group)
- Deltoid
- Gastrocnemius
- Gluteal, External Oblique
- Piriformis
- Pronator Teres
- Psoas Major
- Pyrimidalis
- Quadriceps (group)
- Rectus Abdominus,
- Pyrimidalis
- Soleus
- Trapezius

www.ingramcontent.com/pod-product-compliance
Lightning Source LLC
LaVergne TN
LVHW051055210926
848486LV00002B/113
* 9 7 9 8 9 9 0 1 1 4 1 4 2 *